Je. N. Bilalov

Glaucoma

Je. N. Bilalov

Glaucoma

Educational and methodological manual for teachers of higher medical educational institutions in ophthalmology

ScienciaScripts

Imprint
Any brand names and product names mentioned in this book are subject to trademark, brand or patent protection and are trademarks or registered trademarks of their respective holders. The use of brand names, product names, common names, trade names, product descriptions etc. even without a particular marking in this work is in no way to be construed to mean that such names may be regarded as unrestricted in respect of trademark and brand protection legislation and could thus be used by anyone.

Cover image: www.ingimage.com

This book is a translation from the original published under ISBN 978-620-6-16082-3.

Publisher:
Sciencia Scripts
is a trademark of
Dodo Books Indian Ocean Ltd. and OmniScriptum S.R.L publishing group

120 High Road, East Finchley, London, N2 9ED, United Kingdom
Str. Armeneasca 28/1, office 1, Chisinau MD-2012, Republic of Moldova, Europe
Printed at: see last page
ISBN: 978-620-6-03205-2

GLAUCOMA

Training and methodological manual
for teachers in medical higher education institutions
on the technology of teaching practical ophthalmology classes
to students of medicine and prevention

UDC 617.7:617.7-007.681
LBC
У91

Compilers:

Bilalov E.N. - Doctor of Medicine, Professor, Head of the Department of Ophthalmology, Tashkent Medical Academy.

Nozimov A.E. - PhD, Assistant Professor in the Department of Ophthalmology at the Tashkent Medical Academy.

O.I. Oripov. - PhD, Assistant Professor in the Department of Ophthalmology at the Tashkent Medical Academy.

Reviewers:

S.S. Agzamova - D., Associate Professor, Department of Ophthalmology, Tashkent State Institute of Dentistry.

Narzikulova K.I. - D., Associate Professor, Department of Ophthalmology, Tashkent Medical Academy.

The manual is intended for teachers of medical universities on the technology of training for practical training of students of medical and preventive medicine faculty on the subject of ophthalmology "Glaucoma". This manual is written in accordance with the educational standard and the curriculum of the specialty 5510300 - Medical and preventive medicine.

In addition to the general guidelines that should be followed when presenting theoretical material and teaching practical skills, this manual contains the goals and objectives of the practical session, the necessary knowledge and skills of the student, a lesson planner, situational tasks, tests, control questions, topics of independent work, handouts and used literature.

The teaching manual was considered at a meeting of the Central Teaching and Methodological Council (Minutes No. 6 of 14 February 2023) and approved by the Academic Council of the Tashkent Medical Academy (Minutes No. 8 of 27 February 2023).

Address: 2, Farabi str., Tashkent, Almazar district, 100109.
Tel.: +(998-78) 150-95-09

INTRODUCTION

The work of the health and education systems
as parts of a whole is an important factor in public health.
"Medicine and education are a bridge to justice
between the state and the people"
Mirziyoyev Sh.M.

As a result of reforms over the past five years, the political, legal, socio-economic and scientific-educational foundations necessary for the building of a New Uzbekistan have been created in the country.

In order to further accelerate efforts to promote healthy lifestyles among the population, introduce best practices for early detection and treatment of diseases, and in accordance with Decree No. UP-6035 of 25 July 2020 of President Mirziyoyev on improvement of the system of sanitary and epidemiological well-being and protection of public health, the main areas for medical prevention have been identified, which include the creation of a favourable environment (improvement of the environmental, working, living and living conditions).

The year 2023 has been declared by the head of state as the "Year of Caring for Man and Quality Education". He said that our most precious treasure is our creative people.

The rapid development of medical science, the development and introduction of new technologies into clinical practice and the rapid expansion of the range of medical services determine a steady increase in the quality requirements for medical graduates capable of providing professional assistance to the population at a high level.

The introduction of new state educational standards in higher education institutions implies a transition to innovative learning, as well as new ways of assessing students' learning outcomes. The task of managing the quality of specialist training, including the improvement of objective methods of assessing the knowledge of students and specialist doctors, remains one of the key tasks in the process of their training.

The purpose of teaching ophthalmology in medical school is to equip future physicians with the knowledge, skills and abilities to apply them in medical practice for the diagnosis and treatment of common eye diseases. The discipline of ophthalmology will help you learn how to prevent eye complications from common somatic diseases and eye injuries, as well as eye injuries in mass casualty areas.

This educational and methodical manual, compiled on the basis of the State educational standard, standard and working programs in the direction of medical and preventive medicine (5510300) on the discipline "Ophthalmology" includes, analysis of theoretical and practical part of this lesson. Control of students' knowledge on this topic is carried out with the use of problematic situations, with application of new pedagogical technologies, tests, which are considered as components of problematic learning in different forms (oral, written, independent work of student, etc.). All forms of control are based on the following principles: consistency, regularity, mass coverage of students, objectivity of assessment, etc. This raises the need to choose the best objective method of assessing students' knowledge, which requires reliability of control (survivability), unloading the teacher and improving the quality of control.

In connection with this, developed by the staff of the department teaching-methodical manual, designed for teachers of medical universities, with the aim of training bachelor students in the direction of medical and preventive business (5510300) in the discipline "Ophthalmology" basic knowledge of the subject, necessary in practical activity of future doctors is relevant and timely. It will help future specialists to correctly assess eye symptoms in general diagnosis, to master the rules of hygienic care for the visual organ, to carry out activities necessary for the preservation of the visual organ from various damages, in order to prevent blindness and amblyopia among the population of the republic.

Thus, the use of this manual by teachers in the teaching process will increase the level of mastery of the discipline and therefore improve the quality of the training of future doctors in the field of prevention and medicine.

Authors

GLAUCOMA

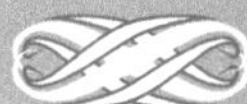

LESSON PREPARATION AND LEARNING OBJECTIVE

Place of the session: classroom, diagnostic room.

Class equipment: teaching aids, teaching materials, case histories, handouts, thematic patients, standard steps and technical equipment for performing practical skills, moulages, Maklakov tonometer, ophthalmoscopes, gonioscope, slit lamp.

Class duration: 240 min.

The aim of the lesson: in the structure of eye pathology glaucoma is one of the most severe diseases leading to incurable blindness and disability. Therefore, the study of research methods used in this pathology, the diagnosis of different forms of primary, secondary glaucoma, the ability to correctly diagnose and treat an acute attack of glaucoma, early diagnosis, prevention and treatment of glaucoma is the purpose of this session.

Objectives:

- Study the circulation of aqueous humour, the structure of the drainage system of the eye;
- To familiarise students with the etiology, pathogenesis, and clinics of closed-angle, open-angle and congenital glaucoma;
- break down the classification schemes for glaucoma;
- to familiarise students with the criteria for diagnosing glaucoma;
- to break down the main treatments for glaucoma;
- to dissect the differential diagnosis of an acute glaucoma attack with acute iridocyclitis;
- To familiarise students with the emergency care of patients with an acute attack of glaucoma;
- to familiarise students with glaucoma early detection, prevention and medical check-ups.

The student should know:

- the features of the clinical picture of glaucoma depending on the stages of the disease;
- basic methods of glaucoma diagnosis;
- indications for conservative, surgical and laser treatment of glaucoma;

• the management of patients with an acute attack of glaucoma;

• the main groups of medicines used in the treatment of glaucoma and their mechanism of action;

• principles for early detection of glaucoma, prevention and screening.

The student should be able to:

• measure the intraocular pressure by palpation;

• be able to conduct a clinical examination using the necessary practical skills;

• make the differential diagnosis of an acute glaucoma attack with acute iridocyclitis;

• give first aid to a patient with an acute attack of glaucoma.

• be able to carry out your own glaucoma prophylaxis.

Motivation.

Glaucoma is one of the most common causes of amblyopia, blindness and disability. Future doctors in their practice will be constantly confronted with the problem of glaucoma. According to the results of mass preventive examinations, among healthy people aged 40 years and older the disease occurs in 12% of cases. The social significance of glaucoma becomes evident when one considers that high morbidity and cases of blindness are noted among people over 40 years of age, among whom the most qualified workers, collective farmers and intellectuals prevail.

The problem of successfully combating glaucoma blindness goes beyond the scope of ophthalmologists and is a general medical task. For this reason, doctors of all specialties must be aware of the signs of the disease, especially the early signs, and be able to refer to a specialist in good time. It is the duty of doctors of all specialties to participate in active preventive examinations that promote early detection and treatment, thus preventing blindness from glaucoma.

Discussing this topic will enable students to learn the main signs of glaucoma, its early detection and prevention.

Inter- and intrasubject links.

Students' knowledge of the topic should cover sufficient skills in related disciplines that correspond to 'horizontal and vertical' integration.

The topic integrates vertically with anatomy in its section 'anatomy of the visual organ', with physiology in its section 'physiology of the visual organ', with histology in its sections 'ontogeny and histology of the visual organ', with deontology in the relationship between patients and staff and with the history of medicine, including the history of ophthalmology.

Horizontally, ophthalmology is integrated with:

- Infectious pathologies, including coronavirus infection and their possible complications on the visual analyser;

- with internal diseases (arterial hypertension, diseases of the gastrointestinal tract, blood, liver and kidneys and various other diseases);

- with endocrinology (diabetes mellitus, hypo- and hyperthyroidism, pituitary and adrenal gland diseases).

- with pharmacology (pharmacotherapy in ophthalmology).

A LIST OF QUESTIONS TO BE DISCUSSED WITH THE STUDENTS DURING THE PRACTICAL SESSION. (General guidelines)

After checking the students present, the teacher formulates the aim of the session and the objectives to be achieved. The teacher gives a definition of glaucoma.

The students' baseline knowledge is then monitored by means of a programmed knowledge test.

The main method of controlling the students' preparation for the lesson is a debriefing session. By actively involving and taking turns questioning the students present, the topic of the lesson is dealt with in detail. The drainage system and the circulation of aqueous humour. Intraocular pressure and the factors determining it. Boundaries of normal intraocular pressure. Diurnal variations of intraocular pressure. True and tonometric pressure. Mechanisms of regulation of intraocular pressure. Modern classification of glaucoma. Principles of glaucoma treatment, prevention and dispensary.

The discussion of the topic of the lesson is conducted using a presentation, showing videos. The discussion of the topic of the lesson is focused on the issues reflected in the lesson plan, control questions. Practical skills are practiced in the course of attending patients and independent work of students with ophthalmic equipment. During the clinical analysis, attention is paid to the deontological features of care in the eye hospital.

The topic is reinforced by interactive learning activities (business games), including case studies and quizzes.

A chronological map of the training session

№	Stages of the session	Forms of exercise	Duration in minutes
			240
1	Introduction by the teacher (rationale for the topic).	The teacher outlines the purpose and flow of the lesson.	10
2	Discussion of homework, Detailed breakdown of the topic by questioning.	The students' initial knowledge level is monitored by means of a programmed quiz. Questioning in the course of the topic analysis.	30

3	Examination of the subject patient in hospital in collaboration with the teacher.	Explains the plan and methodology for the examination of the case patients. The examination of the case is carried out.	40
4	Mastering practical skills. Improving practical skills, working with moulages, ophthalmic equipment.	Palpatory IOP examination, ophthalmoscopy, biomicroscopy, perimetry.	50
5	Discuss the practical part of the lesson.	Questioning, explaining.	20
6	Discussion on the topic of the lesson. Checking the independent work.	Presentation, evaluation, comments and observations, discussion.	40
7	Group work. Demonstration of a video on the topic, analysis of questions, situational tasks, tests, business games, etc.	Demonstration, interactive forms of learning. Assessment by solving situational tasks.	40
8	Conclusion of the trainer on the lesson.	At the end of the lesson, the teacher assesses whether the students have achieved their objectives, points out any mistakes made and how to correct them; names the topic, objectives and course of the next lesson and the required literature for self-study.	10
Total:			240

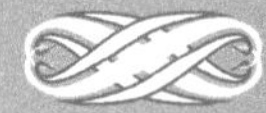

THEORETICAL PART

THE CONTENT AND FLOW OF THE SESSION

GLAUCOMA

After checking on the students present, the teacher formulates the aim of the session, setting specific objectives to be achieved in the session. The teacher then conducts a programmed test control.

The primary programmed control test allows you to assess the initial level of knowledge on the topic. The teacher directs the students' attention to the questions that cause difficulties in their self-study. Topic questions are dealt with by quizzing all the students present. The basic questions of the topic are the control questions of the class:

- the definition of glaucoma;
- the structure of the drainage system of the eye;
- peculiarities of intraocular fluid circulation, outflow pathways;
- intraocular pressure;
- stages in the pathogenesis of the main types of glaucoma ;
- glaucoma optic neuropathy ;
- The main types of glaucoma. Classification;
- risk factors in the development of closed angle, open angle glaucoma;
- clinical manifestations of glaucoma depending on the stage of the process ;
- acute glaucoma attack, mechanism of development, clinic, diagnosis, treatment;
- the sequence of visual field changes in glaucoma patients;
- normal pressure glaucoma, clinic, treatment;
- secondary glaucoma. Mechanisms of development, clinic, treatment;
- Congenital glaucoma. Diagnosis, principles of surgical treatment;
- pharmacotherapy for glaucoma;
- indications for surgical treatment. Basic principles of glaucoma surgery, laser glaucoma surgery;
- glaucoma screening and prevention.

In the introduction, the teacher defines the term 'Glaucoma', indicates the social significance of the problem and clarifies the place of this pathology in the general structure of visual impairment.

Glaucoma (from Greek - colour of sea water, azure) is a severe eye disease that is named after a greenish coloring of the dilated and fixed pupil at the stage of the highest development of the disease process - an acute attack of glaucoma. Glaucoma is a chronic eye disease characterized by a constant or periodic increase in the intraocular pressure (IOP) above the tolerance level due to the outflow of intraocular fluid (IOP) due to the development of trophic disorders in the outflow pathways, progressive optical neuropathy and visual impairment up to irreversible blindness.

Glaucoma can occur at any age from birth, but the prevalence of the disease increases significantly in old age and old age. The incidence of congenital glaucoma is 1 per 10-20 thousand newborns. The primary incidence of glaucoma at the age of 40-45 is around 0.1% of the population, with a prevalence of 1.5% in the 50-60 year age group and over 3% in the 75+ age group. It is one of the leading causes of untreatable blindness and is of major social importance.

The teacher will then ask 2 to 3 students about **the anatomy and physiology of the outflow pathways, pointing out** their importance in the pathogenesis and diagnosis of glaucoma.

The eye cavity contains light-conducting media: aqueous humour filling its anterior and posterior chambers, lens and vitreous body. Regulation of metabolism in the intraocular structures, in particular in the optical media, and maintenance of the eyeball tone is provided by the circulation of aqueous humor in the eye chambers.

Aqueous humour or aqueous humour is an important source of nutrition for the internal structures of the eye. The aqueous humour circulates predominantly in the anterior segment of the eye. It is involved in the metabolism of the lens, cornea, trabecular system, vitreous body and plays an important role in maintaining a certain level of intraocular pressure (IOP). The aqueous humour is continuously produced by the ciliary body appendages. Two mechanisms of IOP production are known:

1. ***The secretory mechanism*** (75%), which is carried out by the pump-metabolic function of the epithelium of the ciliary body's appendages.
2. ***Filtration mechanism*** (25%), especially ultrafiltration (preventing the normal escape of large plasma protein molecules from the capillaries). This mechanism depends entirely on the difference in hydrostatic and oncotic pressures on opposite sides of the membrane structures, i.e. inside the vessel (in blood plasma) and outside it, in chamber moisture.

Circulation of aqueous moisture. The aqueous humour accumulates in the posterior chamber, which is a slit-shaped space with a complex configuration behind the iris. Most of the aqueous humectant then flows out through the pupil, washing around the lens, before entering the anterior chamber and passing through the drainage system of the eye, located in the angle zone of the anterior chamber. The aqueous humour seeps through the trabecular meshwork and collects in the splenic canal, and then drains through 25-30 thin collector tubules (outlets) flowing into the episcleral veins (water veins) of the eye, which are the final point of outflow of aqueous humour.

The described pathway ***(transtrabecular pathway)*** is the main pathway and on average 85-95% of aqueous humour escapes through it. About 15% of aqueous humor escapes from the eye, seeping through the ciliary body stroma and sclera into uveal and scleral veins - ***uveoscleral outflow pathway***. There is a certain equilibrium between the inflow and outflow of HLH. If it is disturbed for some reason, it leads to a change in the IOP level. If the intraocular pressure rises persistently and for a long time, obstacles (blocks) occur, which lead to interference between the eye cavities or closure of the drainage canals. These blocks can be transient (temporary) or organic (permanent).

Students' attention is drawn to the structure of the drainage system and its role in the diagnosis of glaucoma.

The drainage system is located in the corner of the anterior chamber. The peripheral part of the anterior chamber is called the anterior chamber angle (AAC). The anterior wall of the AAC is formed by the corneoscleral junction, the posterior wall by the iris root, and the apex by the ciliary body. There are wide, medium wide, narrow, slit-shaped, and closed AAC. The drainage system of the eye consists of the ***trabecular apparatus*** (TA), the ***scleral sinus*** (Schlemm's canal) and ***the collecting tubules.*** The TA is a net-like ring formed by connective tissue plates with many openings and slits. The TA is a self-cleaning filter that allows one-way fluid movement from the anterior chamber to the scleral sinus. The Schlemm's canal is a circular slit lined with endothelium and located in the posterior outer part of the inner scleral sulcus. There are 25 to 30 collecting tubules (venules) departing from the Schlemm's canal, through which the CSF enters the venous plexus located in the sclera, from which it enters the anterior ciliary veins.

The state of the drainage system of the eye can be assessed using a special examination method - gonioscopy. ***Gonioscopy*** is a method of examining the angle of the anterior chamber, which is performed using a gonioscope and slit lamp. Gonioscopy determines the width of the AAC, as well as the condition of the trabecular tissue and the splenic canal. Different clinical forms of glaucoma are distinguished by gonioscopy. In open-angle glaucoma, all details of the AAC are visible gonioscopically; in closed-angle glaucoma, details of the angle are hidden from view.

The instructor takes apart the intraocular pressure with the students.

Intraocular pressure. IOP (ophthalmotonus) refers to the pressure exerted by the contents of the eyeball on the walls of the eye. The value of IOP is determined by the ratio of a number of factors:

- blood flow and resistance of the intraocular vessels;
- The product and the outflow of aqueous moisture;
- the volume of the lens and the vitreous body;
- the elasticity of the outer membrane - the sclera and cornea.

The teacher points out the physiological role of intraocular pressure and the principles of tonometry.

The physiological role of intraocular pressure is that it maintains the spherical shape of the eyeball and the correct topographic relationship of its internal structures, as well as supports metabolic processes in these structures and the removal of metabolic products from the eye. The relative constancy of the IOP level is regulated and controlled by the hypothalamus and the autonomic nervous system.

The measurement of ophthalmotonus is called ocular ***tonometry.*** The tonometer squeezes and raises the IOP at the moment of measurement. A distinction is therefore made between tonometric and true eye pressure. In tonometry, only the tonometric pressure (Pt) is measured directly. The true ophthalmotonus (Po) is calculated from the tonometric data indirectly or measured with special tonometers.

The McLakov applanation tonometers used in Russia and in our Republic are used to determine the tonometric pressure (Pt). Norms for ***a Maklakov tonometer*** weighing 10 g. - 17 - 26 mmHg. The ***Goldman*** Applanation ***Tonometer*** and ***non-contact pneumotonometer*** readings correspond to true IOP (Po). The normal level of true IOP ranges from 9 to 21 mmHg.

Causes and mechanisms of glaucoma. Glaucoma is classified as a multifactorial disease with a threshold effect. This means that a number of causes are necessary for the development of the disease, and all these combine to make it happen. Of particular importance are heredity, individual characteristics or anomalies in the structure of the eye, and pathology of the cardiovascular, nervous, and endocrine systems.

During the breakdown, the teacher reiterates the importance of knowing the main stages in the development of the pathological process in glaucoma.

The main stages in the development of the pathological process in glaucoma can be represented as follows:

1. The outflow of aqueous humour from the eyeball cavity is disturbed and impaired, which can be due to a multitude of different causes;
2. Increase in intraocular pressure (IOP) above a level that is tolerable for the eye;

3. Deterioration of blood circulation in the tissues of the eye;

4. Hypoxia (lack of oxygen) and ischaemia (impaired blood supply) of the tissue in the optic nerve outlet area;

5. Compression of nerve fibres in the area where they exit the eyeball, resulting in impaired function and death;

6. Dystrophy (malnutrition), degeneration (destruction) and atrophy of optic fibres, disintegration of their maternal retinal ganglion cells;

7. Development of so-called glaucoma optic neuropathy and subsequent optic atrophy (death).

Depending on the severity of the glaucoma process, some of the optic nerve fibres atrophy and some are in a state of parabiosis (a kind of "sleep"), so that their function can be restored by treatment (medication or surgery).

Hydrodynamic block - a marked disturbance of the circulation of the BB in the eye or drainage system of the eye - is the main cause of elevated IOP in glaucoma.

The following variants of the hydrodynamic unit are distinguished:

- incomplete embryonic development of the CPC (CPC dysgenesis);
- pupillary block;
- CPC blockage by the iris root;
- CPC blockage by goniosynechias;
- vitreochristal block;
- trabecular block;
- Schlemm's canal blockage;
- canalicular unit.

Dysgenesis of the AAC causes congenital primary glaucoma, the next 4 types of block are typical for primary and secondary closed angle glaucoma, the last 3 for open angle glaucoma.

The structure of the optic nerve head and its changes in glaucoma are discussed.

The optic nerve head in normal and glaucoma. The optic nerve head (ONH) includes its intraocular part and the section of nerve adjacent to the eye (1-3 mm in length), the blood supply of which depends to some extent on the level of IOP. The GZN consists of retinal ganglion cell axons, astroglia, vessels and connective tissue. The number of nerve fibers in the optic nerve varies from 700,000 to 1,200,000.

The term optic disc (DP) is used to refer to the part of the GZN visible on ophthalmoscopy. A distinction is made between the neural (neuroretinal) ring and the central depression, a physiological excavation in which there is a fibroglial band containing the central retinal vessels. In the area of the passage of the optic nerve, the internal layers of the sclera form the lamina, through which the axons of the retinal ganglion cells pass, forming the disc and the optic nerve trunk. The lamina of the sclera consists of several perforated connective tissue sheets. The perforations form 200 to 400 tubules, with a bundle of nerve fibres passing through each of them.

Glaucoma optic neuropathy (GON) is a major link in the pathogenesis of glaucoma, as its onset and development is a direct cause of visual impairment and blindness in glaucoma patients. Mechanical pressure on the GZN, and ischaemia are the triggering factors leading to the development of GON. Changes in visual function in glaucoma occur unnoticed by the patient and progress slowly. This makes early detection of GON and the differential diagnosis of glaucoma and benign ophthalmic hypertension difficult.

The teacher then details the classification of glaucoma.

Classification of glaucoma. Glaucoma is classified:

by origin - into **primary** and **secondary;**

according to the age of the patient - ***congenital***, ***infantile***, ***juvenile*** and ***adult glaucoma;***

in the mechanism of IOP elevation, ***open-angle***, ***closed-angle***, ***anterior chamber angle dysgenesis***, ***pre-trabecular***, and ***peripheral block;***

IOP is ***hypertensive*** and ***normotensive;***

the degree of GZN damage - ***initial***, ***advanced***, ***far advanced*** and ***terminal;***

according to the course of the disease - ***stabilised*** and ***unstabilised***.

Clinical manifestations of glaucoma depending on the stage of the process. The stage of glaucoma is defined by the visual field and the condition of the DZN. Each stage is indicated by a Roman numeral to briefly record the diagnosis.

The classification of glaucoma identifies 4 stages:

I - Initial;

II - development;

III is far-reaching;

IV - terminal.

The most important diagnostic sign of glaucoma is changes in the visual field. These defects are earliest detected in the central regions and are manifested by a widening of the blind spot and the appearance of arch-shaped protrusions. These disturbances are detected in the early stages of glaucoma, with special visual field examinations. As a rule, patients themselves do not notice these changes in everyday life.

With further development of the glaucomatous process, peripheral visual field defects are detected. The narrowing of the visual field occurs predominantly on the nasal side, with further narrowing of the visual field concentrically covering the peripheral areas until it is completely lost. Dark adaptation is impaired. These symptoms are accompanied by a persistent increase in intraocular pressure (IOP). A drop in visual acuity indicates a severe, advanced stage of the disease, accompanied by almost complete atrophy of the optic nerve.

I - Initial stage. The boundaries of the visual field are normal, but there are slight changes in the paracentral parts of the visual field. Ophthalmoscopically, a widening of the physiological excavation of the DZN can be seen; the ratio of excavation to DZN area does not exceed 0.6.

II - advanced stage. The advanced stage is characterized by narrowing of the peripheral visual field by more than 10 degrees in the superior nasal segment (does not reach 15 degrees from the fixation point); arc-shaped paracentral scotomas in the Bjerrum zone, which are detectable by kinetic perimetry; Glaucomatous excavation of the fundus, 0.6 - 0.8, has a marginal character on the fundus.

Concentric narrowing of the visual field (in the upper nasal segment up to 15 degrees or less from the fixation point, can reach to the centre, closing it), multiple scotomas in the central visual field. Ophthalmoscopy reveals a marginal subtotal excavation of the TZN - 0.8 - 0.9.

IV - terminal stage. Complete loss of vision or retained light perception with irregular projection. Sometimes a small islet of the visual field remains in the temporal sector. On the fundus, there is a total excavation of the DZN with complete destruction of the neuroretinal belt and characteristic displacement of the vascular bundle.

The following gradations of IOP are used when making the diagnosis:

A - IOP within normal values Pt<27 mmHg (Ro<22 mmHg);

B - moderately elevated IOP Pt<33 mmHg (Ro < 33 mmHg);

C - high pressure Pt>32 mmHg (Ro > 32 mmHg).

The features of etiology, pathogenesis, clinic, diagnosis of primary glaucoma are discussed.

Adult primary glaucoma is the most common type of glaucoma associated with age-related changes in the eye. Primary glaucoma is divided into three main clinical forms: ***open angle glaucoma***, ***closed angle glaucoma***, and ***mixed glaucoma.***

Primary open-angle glaucoma is a genetically determined disease characterised by persistent or intermittent elevation of IOP as a result of abnormal outflow of IOP through a pathologically altered drainage system of the eye. In this form of glaucoma, the anterior chamber angle is open.

Etiopathogenesis. There are 3 main pathogenetic mechanisms underlying the pathogenesis of POAG: hydrodynamic, hemocirculatory, and metabolic. The main cause of IOP elevation in glaucoma is hydrodynamic block (impaired outflow of IOP from the eye through the drainage system) resulting from trabeculopathy (dystrophic changes in the trabecular apparatus). Elevated IOP results in deformation of two mechanically weak structures of the eye - the trabecular drainage diaphragm and the scleral lamina. Outward displacement of the trabecular diaphragm leads to a blockage of the sclamus canal, while backward displacement of the scleral plate leads to impingement of the optic nerve fibers in its deformed tubules (SDF excavation).

Risk factors. Heredity, old age, impaired glucocorticoid metabolism, arterial hypotension, diabetes mellitus, impaired pigment metabolism (pigment dispersion syndrome).

Clinic. In most cases of open angle glaucoma, it develops unnoticed by the patient, who does not experience any discomfort, and consults a doctor at a late stage of the disease when he notices a deterioration of visual acuity. A complaint of repeated blurring of vision, iridescent circles around light sources (in the case of 15-20% of patients), heavy eye pain and reddening of the eye are also common. These are the symptoms that occur with an increase in intraocular pressure (IOP) and may be accompanied by pain in the brow and head. Open-angle glaucoma usually affects both eyes, in most cases running asymmetrically.

Ophthalmological status:

- persistent or intermittent elevation of IOP above 26 mmHg (no symptom in normotensive glaucoma);
- the visual field corresponding to the stage of the glaucomatous process;
- Biomicroscopy - dystrophic changes in iris, lens;
- gonioscopy - dystrophic changes in the AAC, with the AAC open;
-Ophthalmoscopy - glaucomatous excavation of the DZN corresponding to the stage of the glaucomatous process.

One type of open-angle glaucoma is ***normal pressure glaucoma***. Glaucoma with normal intraocular pressure has all the typical symptoms of primary glaucoma: changes in the visual field and partial optic atrophy. However, the intraocular pressure remains within the normal range. This type of glaucoma is often combined with a hypotonic type of ophthalmic dystonia.

Primary closed angle glaucoma is characterized by impaired outflow of IAG as a result of anterior chamber angle blocked by the iris root. In this form of glaucoma, the AAC is closed for more than half of its circumference.

Etiopathogenesis. develops in anatomically predisposed eyes with hypermetropia, small eye size, small anterior chamber, large lens, massive iris and ciliary body, more often in eyes with brown iris. Functional factors include increased IOP production, increased blood filling of the intraocular vessels, and dilation of the pupil. Increased IOP is caused by pupillary block, when the pupil is blocked by the large lens and the outflow of IOP from the posterior chamber to the anterior chamber is impaired. The pressure in the posterior chamber increases, the iris shifts forward (bombage) and closes the cPC of the eye.

Clinic. The course of closed angle glaucoma in most patients is characterized by intermittent, initially brief, and then increasingly longer periods of elevated IOP. In the initial stage, this is due to mechanical closure of the trabecular meshwork by the iris root, which is caused by the anatomical predisposition of the eye. The outflow of IOP is reduced. The complete closure of the anterior chamber angle results in a condition called acute attack of closed angle glaucoma. Between attacks, the angle opens. During these attacks, adhesions gradually form between the iris and the anterior chamber angle wall, and the disease gradually becomes chronic with a persistent increase in intraocular pressure (IOP).

In the course of closed angle glaucoma, the phases can be distinguished as follows:

- preglaucoma;
- an acute attack of glaucoma;
- the chronic course of glaucoma.

Preglaucoma occurs in persons who have no clinical manifestations of the disease, but when the anterior chamber angle is examined, it is found to be either narrow or closed. Between pre-glaucoma and an acute attack of glaucoma, transient symptoms of visual discomfort, iridescent circles when looking at a light source, and short-term vision loss may occur. These most commonly occur with prolonged exposure to darkness or emotional arousal (these conditions cause pupil dilation, which fully or partially reduces the outflow of intraocular fluid), and usually disappear on their own, causing little concern to the patient.

The clinical picture of an acute glaucoma attack and the principles of emergency medical care are discussed in detail.

An acute glaucoma attack is triggered by triggering factors such as nervous tension, overexertion, being in the dark for a long time, dilation of the pupil with medication, prolonged work with the head tilted, and taking large quantities of fluids. Sometimes an attack occurs for no apparent reason.

Complaints. The patient complains of pain in the eye and head, blurred vision, and iridescent circles when looking at a light source. The pain is caused by compression of the nerve elements in the iris root and ciliary body. If the attack is severe, nausea and vomiting may occur, and there may be pain radiating to the heart and abdomen, sometimes mimicking a cardiovascular condition.

Ophthalmological status:

- eyelid swelling, narrowing of the eye crevice, congestion in the eye;
- diffuse corneal oedema;
- at the height of the seizure, visual acuity may decrease dramatically;
- shallow front camera (its absence);
- paralytic mydriasis, irregularly shaped pupil, unresponsive to light;

- Biomicroscopy - shallow anterior chamber, iris bombage, iris haemorrhages, iris vessel strangulation followed by aseptic necrosis of the iris stroma;

- IOP> 50 mmHg. - The eye is dense, like a "stone";

- the CPC is closed during gonioscopy (if it is possible to examine it).

If the pressure is not relieved by medication or surgery within hours of an attack developing, the eye is at risk of irreversible vision loss. An acute glaucoma attack is an emergency and requires urgent medical attention.

The differential diagnosis of an acute glaucoma attack is primarily made with general illnesses that occur suddenly and are accompanied by severe headache, nausea and vomiting (food intoxication, hypertensive crisis, acute cerebral circulation disorders).

Treatment of an acute glaucoma attack. During the first hour, instillation of 1% pilocarpine hydrochloride solution every 15 min, then every hour (2 - 4 times) and every 4 hours thereafter. At the same time the affected eye is injected with 0.5% - timolol maleate solution and 2% - azopt solution. Diacarb 0.25 g was administered orally. 2 - 3 times a day, osmotic drugs (urea, glycerin 1 -1.5 g / kg per day), parenterally - 20% mannitol solution intravenously, 1% furosemide solution intravenously or intramuscularly 20 - 40 mg / day. For a prolonged attack a lytic mixture should be used: 1 to 2 ml of 2.5% aminazine solution, 1 ml of 2% dimedrol solution, 1 ml of 2% promedolol solution. After the mixture has been administered, the patient should be in bed for 3 hours.

Distraction therapy (hot foot baths, leeches on the temple) is given at the same time as medication. If the attack cannot be managed within 12-24 hours, surgical treatment - peripheral iridectomy, surgical or laser treatment - is indicated.

The etiopathogenesis and types of secondary glaucoma are discussed.

Secondary glaucoma is a consequence of other ocular or general diseases, accompanied by damage to those ocular structures that are involved in the circulation of intraocular moisture or its outflow from the eye.

A large number of different forms of secondary glaucoma can be grouped into a number of groups, depending on the etiology:

1. Inflammatory and post-inflammatory;
2. Phacogenic (phacotopic, phacomorphic, phacolytic);
3. Vascular;
4. Dystrophic;
5. Traumatic;
6. Post-operative;
7. Neoplastic;
8. Other reasons.

Treatment is symptomatic and the underlying disease is treated at the same time. Hypotensive drugs are prescribed topically. Surgical treatment.

Congenital glaucoma is discussed in detail.

Congenital glaucoma can be genetically determined (predetermined) or caused by disease and trauma in the fetus during embryonic development or during birth. This type of glaucoma manifests itself in the first weeks and months of life, and sometimes several years after birth. It is quite rare (1 case per 10-20 thousand newborns).

Classification:

1. Primary congenital glaucoma.
2. Concomitant congenital glaucoma.

Primary congenital glaucoma includes several varieties:

- congenital glaucoma, or hydrophthalmia (signs of the condition appear in the first year of life);

- Infantile, or delayed, congenital glaucoma (aged 3 - 10 years);

- juvenile glaucoma (11 - 35 years old);

Combined congenital glaucoma occurs with other anomalies and developmental defects in the child.

Congenital glaucoma clinic. The first symptoms are noticed by parents, then specialists become involved. Sometimes congenital glaucoma occurs in utero.

Complaints of photophobia, lacrimation. Intermittent or persistent redness of the eye (symptoms are associated with corneal distension due to enlargement of the eyeball).

Ophthalmological status. Wide pupil - mydriasis, impaired pupil response to light. Increased corneal size>9.0 mm, stromal and epithelial edema, accompanied by loss of corneal transparency and luster. Deepening of the anterior chamber of the eye. Increase of eyeball size in all directions with dystrophic changes in the eyeball - buphthalmus. Increase in IOP. Ocular fundus shows glaucomatous excavation of the DZN, corresponding to the stage of the process. Gonioscopy - dysgenesis of varying severity, sometimes combined with congenital anomalies.

Primary congenital glaucoma (PVG or hydrophthalmos) occurs before the age of 3 years, recessive inheritance (sporadic cases are possible). Pathomechanism - dysgenesis of the AAC and IOP increase, clinical symptoms - photophobia, lacrimation, blepharospasm, enlargement of the eyeball, corneal edema and increase in size, exasculation of the DZN.

Primary infantile glaucoma (PIG) occurs in children aged 3 to 10 years, with the same inheritance and pathomechanisms as PVG. IOP is elevated, corneal and ocular dimensions are unchanged, and the excavation of the DZN increases as the glaucoma progresses.

Primary juvenile glaucoma (PJG) occurs between the ages of 11 and 35 years, heredity is related to abnormalities in chromosome 1 and TIGR, pathomechanisms are trabeculopathy or goniodysgenesis, IOP is elevated, changes in DZN and glaucomal visual function.

Concomitant congenital glaucoma. Glaucoma may be combined with other congenital anomalies: microcornea, sclerocornea, aniridia, persistent primary vitreous, peripheral or central mesodermal dysgenesis (Rieger, Frank-Kamenetsky syndrome, Peters anomaly), homocysteinemia, Marfan syndrome, Marquesani, Lowe syndrome, Sturge-Weber fibromatosis. neurofibromatosis, chromosomal abnormalities.

Treatment. Drug treatment is ineffective and is usually complementary to surgical treatment. Two principles underpin surgical treatment: timeliness and pathogenetic orientation. Surgery must be performed as early as possible, in fact as soon as the diagnosis is made. The choice of the type of surgery is based on the results of gonioscopy. Since all congenital glaucomas are closed-angle, the main principle is to improve the outflow of IHG.

The prevention of congenital glaucoma lies in the prevention of inbreeding, a healthy lifestyle for the pregnant woman, and timely sanitation of chronic infections before and during pregnancy.

For all congenital glaucoma, early surgical treatment (goniotomy, fistulising surgery) performed in the early stages of the disease preserves vision.

Treatment of glaucoma includes hypotensive pharmacotherapy, surgery (laser and surgical), and correction of haemodynamic and metabolic disturbances with medication and physiotherapy.

The methodology of the myotics regimen and the basics of glaucoma medication treatment are discussed, focusing on the importance of their individual selection and the optimal frequency of injection. The importance of regular local and general treatment, a sparing regime of life, diet and work, and regular medical check-ups are emphasised. The indications for surgical treatment of patients are reviewed in detail. The importance of a rational choice of the type of antiglaucoma surgery is emphasised.

Hypotensive pharmacotherapy is carried out with hypotensive drugs, which are divided into two groups according to their effect on the hydrodynamics of the eye:

- agents that inhibit the production of intraocular fluid.
- drugs that improve the anterior and posterior outflow of intraocular fluid;

The first group includes adrenoblockers (timolol maleate, arutimol, betoptic), carbohydrate inhibitors (azopt), combination medicines (photil, photil forte) and osmotic agents (glycerol, mannitol).

The second group of drugs includes: cholinomimetics (pilocarpine), sympathomimetics (epinephrine, dipivefrine) and prostaglandins (xalatan).

Laser and surgical treatment.

Laser treatment for glaucoma is aimed at removing intraocular blocks in the pathway of aqueous humour through the drainage system of the eye. Various types of lasers are used for this purpose, but the most common are argon lasers, pulsed neodymium IAG lasers, as well as diode lasers.

The main point ***of laser iridectomy is*** to form holes in the periphery of the iris. This equalises the pressure in the anterior and posterior chambers, opening the angle of the anterior chamber and restoring the drainage system. ***Laser trabeculoplasty*** is performed for open-angle glaucoma. A series of cauterizations on the inner surface of the trabecular meshwork expands the pores in the trabecular meshwork and improves the inflow of aqueous humour through the drainage system. Cyclodestructive surgery is performed with the laser to reduce aqueous humour production.

If conservative and laser therapies are not effective enough, ***surgical treatment*** is indicated. There is a wide variety of surgical interventions, which can be divided into five main groups:

- operations that improve the circulation of aqueous humour inside the eye;
- fistulizing operations;
- non-penetrating fistulizing surgery;
- operations with the use of glaucoma drains;
- cyclo-destructive surgery.

The teacher draws the students' attention to the principles, stages of glaucoma prevention and dispensation.

Glaucoma screening and prevention.

The follow-up of glaucoma patients involves active and dynamic observation of the condition of the eye, registration of this category of the population with a view to early detection and comprehensive treatment of the disease, measures to improve working and living conditions, prevent the development and spread of disease, restore ability to work and conduct a period of active life.

Monitoring is part of the follow-up measures and is a set of diagnostic methods needed to clarify the extent of glaucoma and the rate of the pathological process. The follow-up of patients should be carried out in ***two stages.***

The first stage involves active identification of patients with glaucoma and risk groups, and monitoring the course of the glaucoma process, which is carried out on the bases of territorial polyclinics, medical clinics and central district hospitals.

Objectives of the first phase:

- Preventive check-ups among the healthy population to identify patients with suspected glaucoma and refer them for in-depth ophthalmological examinations;

- collecting a genealogical anamnesis, working with relatives;
- monitoring of glaucoma patients. Scheduled examinations, referral to coordinating centres for newly detected glaucoma patients, those with decompensated IOP and destabilised glaucoma, and in-depth examinations of all patients once a year and planned courses of anti-dystrophic and neuroprotective treatment.

The second stage is provided in specialised ophthalmology centres, where early diagnosis of glaucoma in patients referred with suspected glaucoma is carried out, as well as treatment measures to stabilise the process.

Objectives of the second phase:

- In-depth examinations of patients using the latest diagnostic techniques for early and preclinical detection of glaucoma;
- dynamic follow-up of people with suspected glaucoma;
- rehabilitation of patients with diagnosed glaucoma (selection of hypotensive drugs, laser and surgical treatment).

Ophthalmologists in polyclinics carry out routine screening of patients with glaucoma. Consultative, diagnostic and therapeutic care is provided in specialised glaucoma centres.

Prevention of blindness and disability from glaucoma includes regular monitoring of intraocular pressure in the population over the age of 40, especially if there is a family history of glaucoma or relatives. It is very important to reestablish glaucoma clinics, which are of great preventive and diagnostic importance.

After reviewing the theoretical material, the teacher demonstrates the Maklakov tonometer and explains the technique of measuring IOP by applanation tonometry and palpation. Introduces the principles of non-contact tonometry and tonography.

Together with the teacher, the students examine patients diagnosed with glaucoma who have been prepared in advance. Particular attention is paid to collecting the anamnesis, clarifying the patient's complaints at the time of treatment, and the students' ability to apply their theoretical knowledge in practice.

A case study is used to demonstrate basic examination techniques, which include visometry, perimetry, ophthalmoscopy, gonioscopy and tonometry. At the end of the patient's examination, a clinical review is carried out with additions and comments.

The students are then asked to solve the situation problems.

The teacher assesses the students' solutions to the case studies. As an option for independent work, the students prepare at home presentations on the topic of the class.

They speak in public, the teacher evaluates the performance and presentation and makes a summary.

The teacher allows time for students to learn and improve their practical skills. Work with moulages, ophthalmic equipment.

Finally, the teacher sums up and gives the task for the next session.

THE USE OF A GRAPHICAL ORGANISER VENN DIAGRAM

Used to compare or contrast or contrast 2-3 aspects and show what they have in common. In this session to make a differential diagnosis between acute glaucoma attack and acute iridocyclitis.

Develops systems thinking, comparison, comparison, analysis and synthesis.

Steps:

1. The students are introduced to the rules of making a Venn Diagram. Individually/p in pairs, draw a Venn Diagram and fill in the parts of the non-overlapping circles (x).
2. Pair up, compare and complete their diagrams.
3. At the intersection of the circles, make a list of those features that they think are common to the information of the two/three circles (xx/xxx).

Острый приступ глаукомы
Острый иридоциклит
• Радужные круги при взгляде на свет;
• Иррадиирующие боли;
• Предшествуют продромальные приступы
• Инъекция передних цилиарных артерий
• Чувствительность роговицы снижена
• Передняя камера мелкая
• Зрачок расширен
• ВГД повышено
Боль, покраснение глаза,снижение зрения
• Радужных кругов нет
• Боли в самом глазу
• Глаз заболевает внезапно
• Перикорнеальная иньекция
• Чувствительность роговицы не изменена
• Передняя камера средней глубины или глубокая
• Зрачок сужен
• ВГД нормальное или снижено

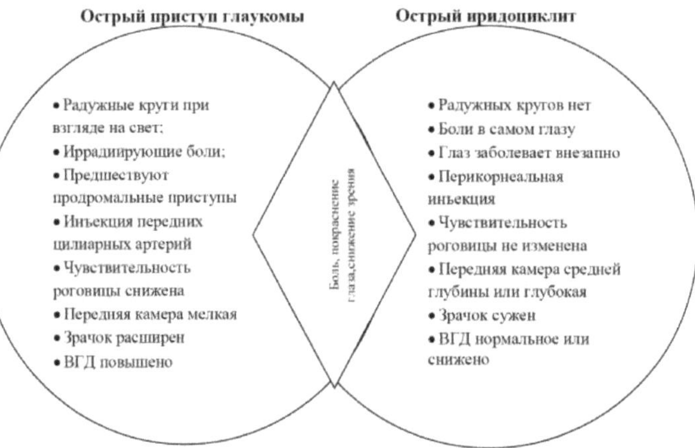

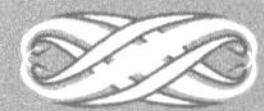

ANALYTICAL PART

Situation tasks:

1. The parents of a 1-year-old child consulted an ophthalmologist regarding an increase in the size of their child's right eye. On examination: the right eyeball is enlarged compared to the left eye, there is an increase in cornea size and swelling, lacrimation. On ophthalmoscopy: optic disc excavation is dilated. The left eye is without pathological changes.

Questions:	**Answers:**
1. Make a diagnosis.	1. Congenital glaucoma, buphthalmus.
2. treatment.	2. operative.
3. the doctor's tactics.	3 Refer your child to a paediatric ophthalmologist a logical hospital.

2. An elderly woman arrived in an emergency. A sudden onset of severe headache with irradiation into the left eye, nausea, vomiting. According to the patient, the vision in this eye had been decreased recently. Pulse rate was slow - 60 beats per minute. BP 170/95 mmHg. On objective examination: moderate narrowing of the left eye slit, redness of the left eye, cornea cloudy, pupil dilated, poorly responding to light. When determining visual acuity there is an abnormal perception of light (lack of subjective vision). Palpatory IOP: +3

Questions:	**Answers:**
1. Presumptive diagnosis.	1. an acute attack of glaucoma in the left eye.
2. First aid.	2. Frequent pilocarpine injections, osmodi uretics, distraction therapy.
3. doctor's tactics	3 Refer the patient to an ophthalmology hospital.

3. A 70-year-old patient O. was admitted in an emergency and complained of severe pain in the left eye. Past medical history: over the last 4 years the vision in the left eye had been gradually decreasing. The patient had only seen light in that eye for the last few months. Pain in this eye occurred for the first time. On examination: mixed injection of the eyeball vessels, corneal edema, anterior chamber shallow, pupil grey, lens cloudy. Visual acuity: light perception with correct light projection. IOP = 40 mmHg.

Questions: **Answers:**

1. Make a diagnosis.	1. Secondary glaucoma, swollen cataract.
2 Determine the doctor's tactics.	2. Referral for surgical treatment.
3. Prevention.	3. the surgical treatment of cataracts.

4. The patient is 51 years old. Right eye is healthy. Left eye: complains of iridescent circles around a light source and fog in front of the eyes in the morning. On examination: IOP 36 mmHg. In spite of 3x pilocarpine 1%, eye functions were worsening, visual acuity 0.3, not corrected, field of vision narrowed by 20 degrees from periphery. Gonioscopically, all elements of the angle are closed by the iris root. Ocular fundus: optic disc pale glaucomatous excavation.

Questions:	**Answers:**
1. Your diagnosis.	1. Closed-angle 2 "c" glaucoma.
2. Recommended treatment.	2. Antiglaucoma surgery needed
3. Differential diagnosis.	3. Cataract

Test questions on the topic

1. Symptoms common to all types of glaucoma:

A. Increase resilience, reduce aqueous outflow
B. Unstable intraocular pressure
C. Increased intraocular pressure levels
D. Changing the field of vision
E. All of the above are true*

2. Symptoms not characteristic of an acute attack of primary closed angle glaucoma:

A. Corneal oedema
B. Shallow front camera
C. Wide, elliptical pupil
D. Congestive injection of the eyeball
E. Pupil narrow, pupil response to light preserved*

3. On the basis of which signs the differential diagnosis of glaucomatous and physiological excavation is made:

A. Excavation values
B. Depths of optic disc excavation *
C. Excavation depths
D. The marginal nature of the excavation
E. All of the above are true.

4. The most relevant for the diagnosis of primary glaucoma is:

A. Daily tonometry
B. Tonography
C. Gonioscopy
D. Field of view study
E. Investigations of the optic disc
F. All of the above*

5. Differential symptom characteristic of acute glaucoma as opposed to acute iridocyclitis:

A. Reddening of the eye
B. Pain
C. Tearfulness
D. The presence of purulent discharge from the eyes
E. Presence of iridescent circles when looking at the light*

6. Commonalities in the course of primary open-angle and closed-angle glaucoma:

A. Progressive deterioration of fluid outflow from the eye
B. Constriction of the pupil
C. Development of glaucomatous optic atrophy *
D. Increased pigmentation of the anterior chamber angle
E. Swelling of the anterior part of the iris.

7. The stages of primary glaucoma are assessed by indicators:

A. Visual acuity
B. Intraocular pressure levels
C. Areas of glaucomatous optic disc excavation
D. States of the visual field *
E. The range of daily fluctuations in IOP.

8. Upper limit of normal intraocular pressure when

measured with the Maklakov tonometer:

A. 20 mmHg;
B. 24 mmHg;
C. 26 mmHg; *.
D. 28 mmHg;
E. There is no single norm.

9. The visual field in the initial stage of primary glaucoma is narrowed from:

A. Up to 45°;
B. Up to 20°;
C. Up to 10°;
D. Up to 5°;
E. Not constricted*.

10. The front camera angle unit can be called up:

A. Unabsorbed mesodermal tissue
B. The root of the iris
C. Newly formed vessels
D. By blood
E. All of the above*

11. The pathogenesis of congenital glaucoma is based on:

A. Incorrect positioning of the anterior chamber angle structures
B. Insufficient differentiation of the corneoscleral trabeculae
C. Presence of mesodermal tissue in the corner of the anterior chamber *
D. Hyperproduction of aqueous humour by the ciliary body
E. Change in the drainage system at the intrascleral level.

12. The leading signs of hydrophthalmus are:

A. Increased size of the cornea
B. Increased size of the eyeball
C. Increased IOP
D. Deep front camera
E. All of the above are true*

13. In the early diagnosis of glaucoma, the most informative ones are:

A. Daily tonometry
B. Tonography
C. Field of view study
D. Biomicroscopy of the anterior segment of the eye
E. Correct all of the above*

14. An unstable glaucomatous process is indicated by:

A. Decreased visual acuity
B. Appearance of pain in the eye
C. Progressive narrowing of the visual field *
D. Expansion of glaucomatous DZN excavation
E. Lack of normalisation of intraocular pressure.

15. The dynamics of the glaucomatous process are characterised by:

A. Intraocular pressure value
B. Value of the ease of outflow coefficient
C. State of the visual field *
D. Condition of the optic disc
E. A change in the shape of the pupil.

16. There are no risk factors for ophthalmic hypertension:

A. Glaucoma patients in the immediate family
B. Ophthalmotonus exceeds 30 mmHg.
C. Cataract changes in the lens *
D. Asymmetry in ophthalmotonus in two eyes

E. Asymmetry in the magnitude of DZN excavation in the two eyes.

17. Ocular hypotensive drug groups:
A. Cholinomimetics
B. Anticholinesterase drugs
C. Beta adrenoblockers
D. Carboanhydrase inhibitors
E. All of the above*

18. Anticholinesterase agents do not include:
A. Ezerin;
B. Armin;
C. Phosphacol;
D. Prostaglandin*
E. Demecarium bromide (tosmilene).

19. Remedies that do not reduce the production of watery moisture:
A. Timolol;
B. Clopheline (clonidine);
C. Emoxipine; *.
D. Acetazolamide (diacarb);
E. Betaxalol (betoptic).

20. Not prescribed for the general treatment of glaucoma:
A. Vasodilators
B. Angioprotectors
C. Corticosteroids *
D. Antioxidants
E. Drugs that improve retinal and optic nerve metabolism.

21. Physiotherapy treatments for glaucomatous atrophy of the DZN do not include:
A. Magnetotherapy
B. Low-energy laser irradiation
C. Electrostimulation
D. Ultraviolet irradiation*
E. UHF.

22. A glaucoma patient's regime provides for everything but:
A. Restrictions on fluid intake
B. Restriction of visual work
C. Avoid working with a prolonged head tilt
D. Excluding physical work
E. Smoking*.

23. Timolol is contraindicated in glaucoma patients with glaucoma:
A. Proclivity to sore throat
B. Bradycardia *
C. Urolithiasis
D. Heart block
E. Dry eye syndrome.

PRACTICAL SKILLS

Note: If a student has fully completed the practical skill step, he/she will receive a score of complete answer. In case of even an incomplete answer, the practical skill step is considered as not completed and is scored as "0" **point**

Determining visual acuity

(assessment criteria for the step-by-step performance of a practical skill)

№	Content of the answer	Points	
		Full answer	No answer or an incomplete answer
1	Need: Roth apparatus, Sivtsev-Golovin table or remote controlled table (phoroptre), pointer	10	0
2	Roth apparatus with a Sivtsev-Holovin table (phoropter) placed at a distance of 5 m from the subject (line 10 of the table should be at eye level of the subject)	10	0
3	Examine each eye separately, with one eye covered by a shutter	10	0
4	Determination of visual acuity begins with showing optotypes of row 10 (vis=1.0), showing them in a breakdown from bottom to top	10	0
5	For people with reduced vision, it is acceptable to start the examination from row 1, showing from top to bottom	10	0
6	Visual acuity is assessed according to the row in which all the signs have been named correctly (row 1 = 0.1; row 2 = 0.2 etc.)	10	0
7	If the patient cannot distinguish between optotypes of line 1, visual acuity is determined using a finger reading and calculated using the Snellen formula d where d is the distance with Vis= --which the patient is un- D indicates the number of fingers of the hand; D = 50 m	20	0
8	In the absence of subject vision, light perception is examined by directing the light. Light perception can be correct and	10	0

	incorrect		
9	In the absence of light perception, visual acuity is "0".	10	0
TOTAL		100	0

Lower and upper eyelid eversion

(assessment criteria for the step-by-step performance of a practical skill)

№	Content of the answer	Points	
		Full answer	No answer or an incomplete answer
1	To examine the lower eyelid, the patient is asked to look up	20	0
2	With the thumb of the right or left hand, pull the skin of the lower eyelid downwards	20	0
3	To examine the upper eyelid, the patient is asked to look down	10	0
4	With the right thumb and left hand, pull the eyelid skin backwards	10	0
5	With the thumb and forefinger of the right hand, pull the eyelid down and to the front	10	0
6	Use the thumb of your left hand to create a skin fold	10	0
7	Press on the cartilage of the upper eyelid and with the right hand bring the upper eyelid upwards	10	0
8	The conjunctiva of the eyelids, the eyeball and the vaults can be examined with this method	10	0
TOTAL		100	0

Palpatory determination of intraocular pressure

(assessment criteria for the step-by-step performance of a practical skill)

№	Content of the answer	Points	
		Full answer	No answer or an incomplete answer
1	Ask the person to close their eyes and look down	20	0
2	Palpatory determination of eye pressure inside by alternating pressure on the eye with the index fingers of both hands	20	0
3	If palpation is slightly fluctuating, IOP is considered normal	20	0

4	If there is no fluctuation, IOP is high (T+1 to T+3)	20	0
5	If palpation shows fluid fluctuation and the fingers seem to "fall" into the eye, then the intraocular pressure is low (T-1 to T-3)	20	0
	TOTAL	100	0

FORMS OF MONITORING KNOWLEDGE, SKILLS AND ABILITIES

- a grade for the oral examination (AE);
- assessment for solving programmed tests (PTs);
- the grade for the situational problem solving (SZ);
- an assessment of the learning of practical skills (SP);
- the assessment of independent work (AW).

The students' total grade for the practical training - current control (TC) is assigned on the basis of the average value of the sum of grades for oral examination (30%), solution of programmed tests (10%) and situational tasks (10%), demonstration of mastered practical skills (40%), as well as for independent work (10%), which is calculated according to the following formula:

$$\mathbf{TC = (YO \times 0.3) + (PT \times 0.1) + (SS \times 0.1) + (NS \times 0.4) + (SS \times 0.1)}$$

Oral assessment criteria

№	Evaluation	Criteria
1.	Great "5"	Has fully grasped the theoretical and methodological concepts of the subject, expresses his/her opinion on the topic, answers all questions correctly, analyses and draws conclusions, thinks creatively, takes an active part in the discussion of the topic in class, has a free imagination and shares his/her opinion with the teacher when necessary.
2.	Good "4"	Has fully grasped the theoretical and methodological concepts of the subject, adequately expresses his/her opinion on the topic, answers not all questions, does analysis and inference, thinks creatively, participates in the discussion of the topic in class, has a clear understanding of the topic of this homework.
3.	Satisfactory "3"	Expresses an opinion on the topic, answers questions incompletely, participates in the discussion of the topic in class, has an understanding of the topic of the given homework.

4.	Unsatisfactory "2"	Cannot express an opinion on the topic, does not answer questions, does not participate in the discussion of the topic in class, does not have an understanding of the topic of this homework

Criteria for assessing students' independent work

№	Evaluation	**Criteria**
1.	Great "5"	Preparation of presentations for independent work (tables, charts, slides) to a high modern level. Solid mastery of the presentation plan for independent work in the practical session in its entirety.
2.	Good "4"	Preparation of presentations for independent work (tables, charts, slides) at a good level. Not fully mastered the plan for the presentation of independent work in the practical session.
3.	Satisfactory "3"	The preparation of presentations for independent work (tables, diagrams, slides) is incomplete. The mastery of the presentation plan for independent work in the practical session is below the required level.
4.	Unsatisfactory "2"	Did not prepare a presentation

Table
on converting a 100-point scale to a 5-point scale

100 point scale	**5 ballroom Evaluation**	**100 point scale**	**5 ballroom Evaluation**	**100 point scale**	**5 ballroom Evaluation**	**100 point scale**	**5 ballroom Evaluation**
86-100	5	71-85	4	55-70	3	<55	2

Questions

1. Definition of glaucoma.
2. The structure of the drainage system of the eye;
3. Features of intraocular fluid circulation, outflow pathways.
4. Intraocular pressure.
5. Stages of pathogenesis of the main types of glaucoma.
6. Glaucoma optic neuropathy.
7. The main types of glaucoma. Classification.
8. Risk factors in the development of closed angle, open angle glaucoma.
9. Clinical manifestations of glaucoma depending on the stage of the

process.

10. Acute glaucoma attack, mechanism of development, clinic, diagnosis, treatment.
11. The sequence of visual field changes in glaucoma patients.
12. Normal pressure glaucoma, clinic, treatment.
13. Secondary glaucoma. Mechanisms of development, clinic, treatment.
14. Congenital glaucoma. Classification.
15. Pharmacotherapy for glaucoma.
16. The basic principles of surgical treatment for glaucoma.
17. Laser glaucoma surgery.
18. Glaucoma screening and prevention.

Topics for students' independent work

1. The structure of the drainage system of the eye.
2. Intraocular pressure.
3. An acute attack of glaucoma.
4. Changes in the visual field in glaucoma.
5. Congenital glaucoma.
6. Glaucoma screening and prevention.

HANDOUTS

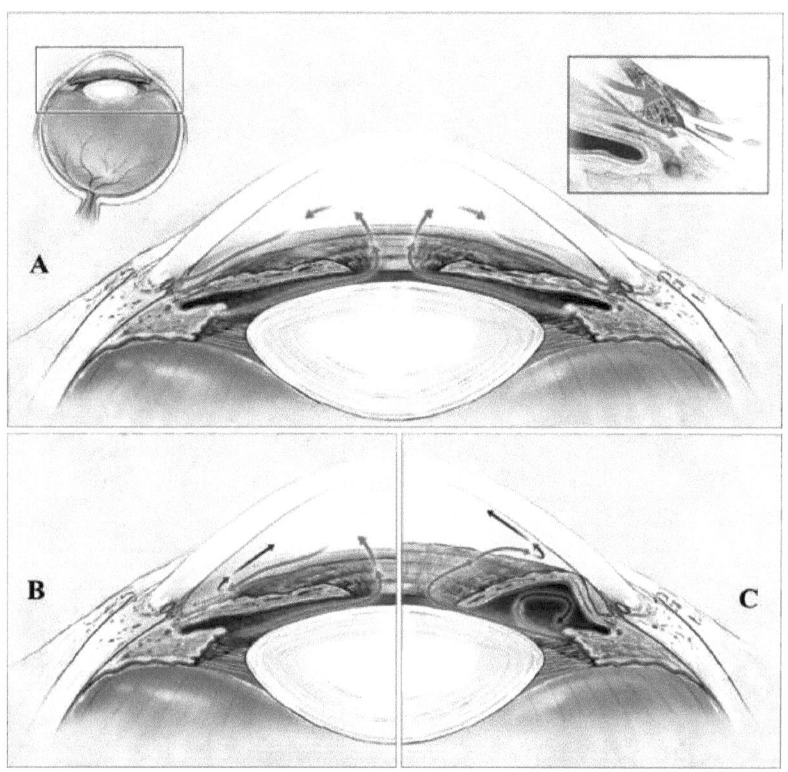

A) Pathways of outflow of intraocular fluid in normal circumstances;
B) In open-angle glaucoma; C) In closed-angle glaucoma

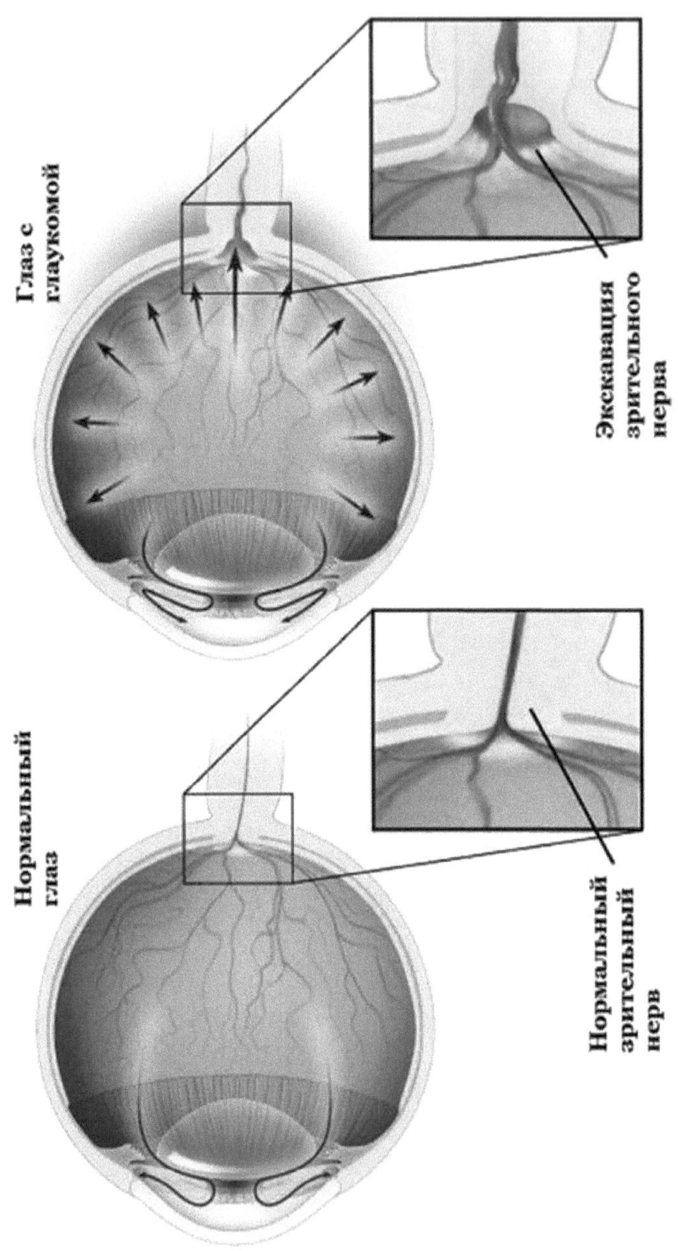
Нормальный глаз
Глаз с глаукомой
Нормальный зрительный нерв
Экскавация зрительного нерва

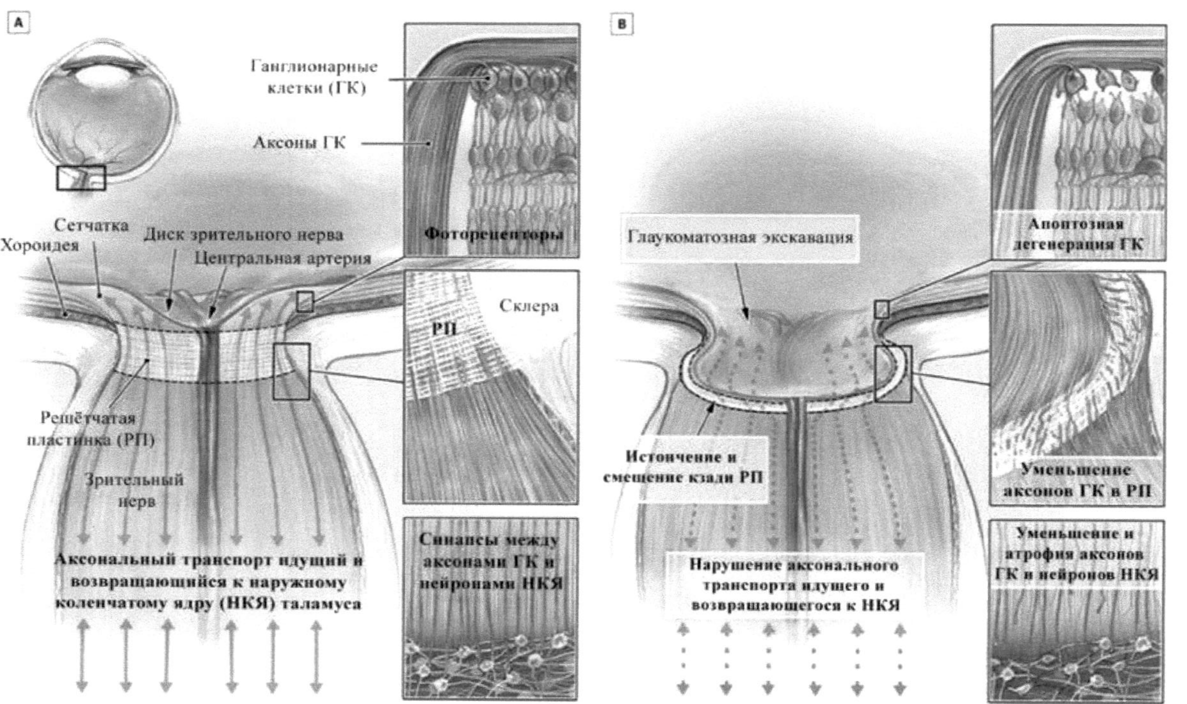

A) Normal anatomy; B) Neurodegenerative changes associated with glaucomatous optical neuropathy

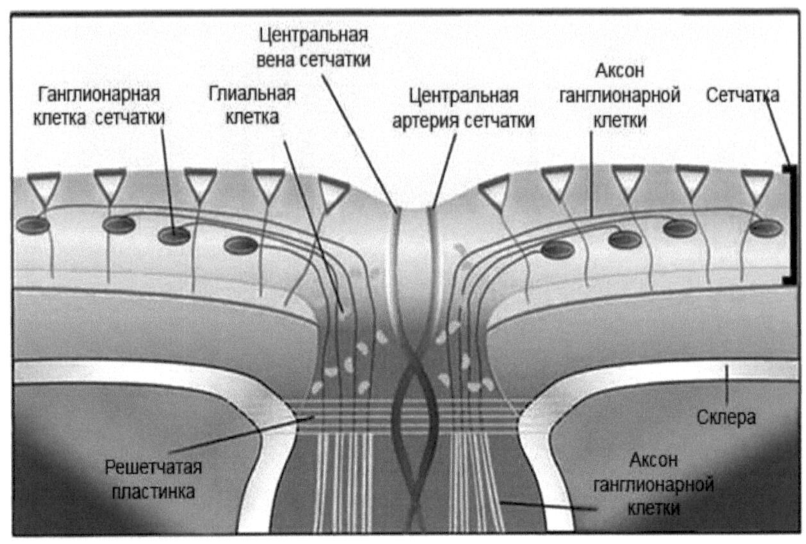
Центральная
вена сетчатки
Ганглионарная
клетка сетчатки
Глиальная
клетка
Центральная
артерия сетчатки
Аксон
ганглионарной
клетки
Сетчатка
Склера
Решетчатая
пластинка
Аксон
ганглионарной
клетки

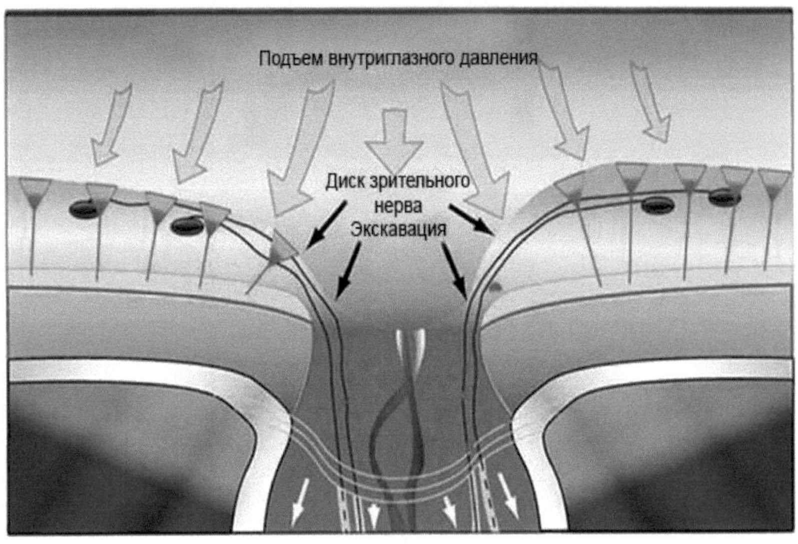
Подъем внутриглазного давления
Диск зрительного
нерва
Экскавация

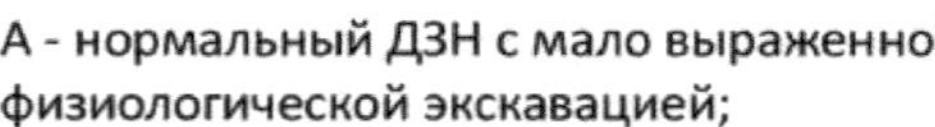

А - нормальный ДЗН с мало выраженной физиологической экскавацией;

Б - концентрическое расширение и увеличение экскавации;

В - нижне-темпоральное смещение зоны экскавации и штрихообразные гемморагии по краю диска свидетельствуют о прогрессировании глаукомы;

Г - дальнейшее прогрессирование глаукомы;

Д - субтотальная экскавация;

Е - тотальная экскавация

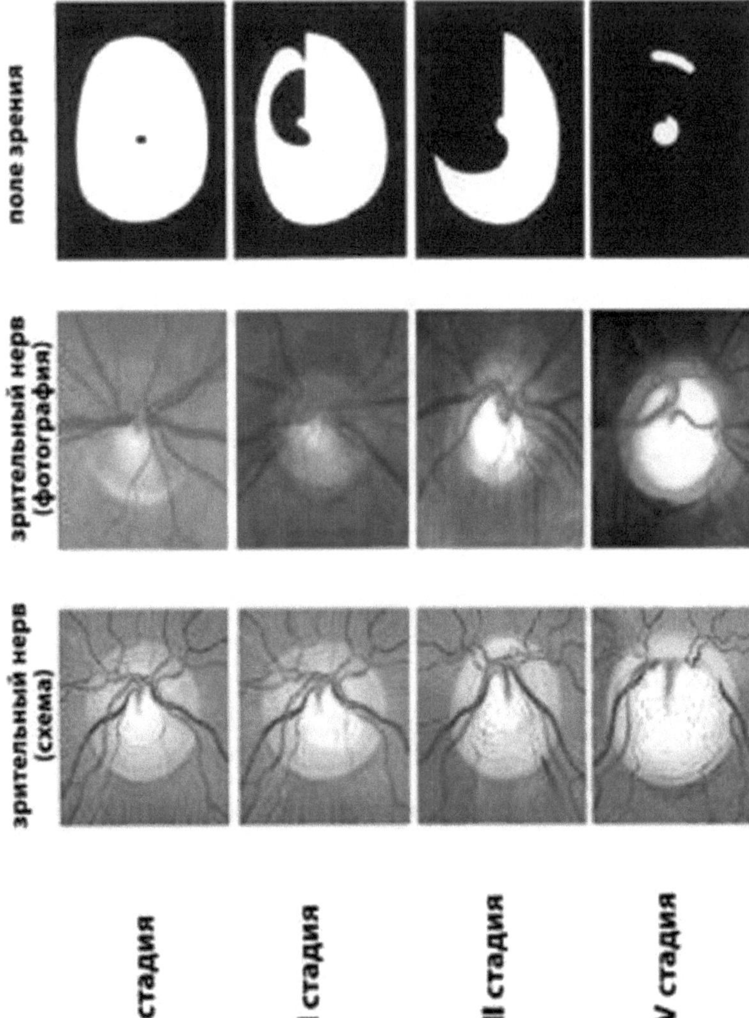
поле зрения
зрительный нерв (фотография)
зрительный нерв (схема)
I стадия
II стадия
III стадия
IV стадия

Исследование поля зрения

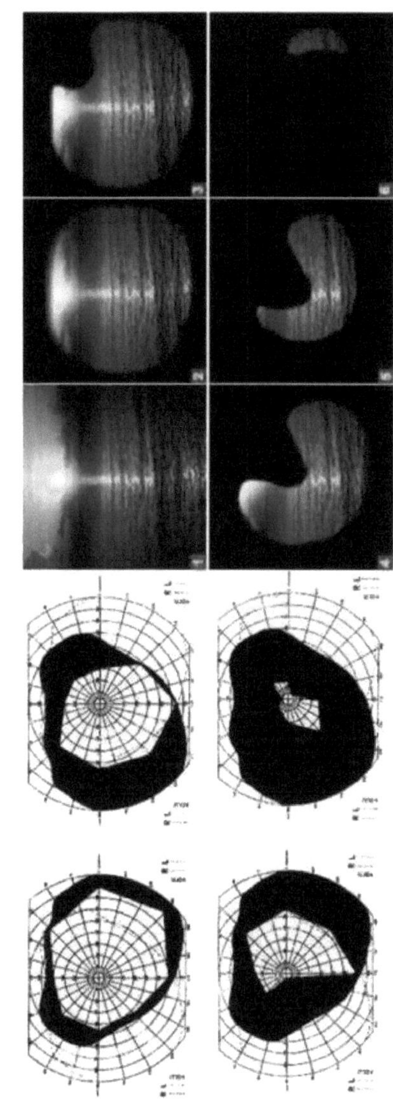

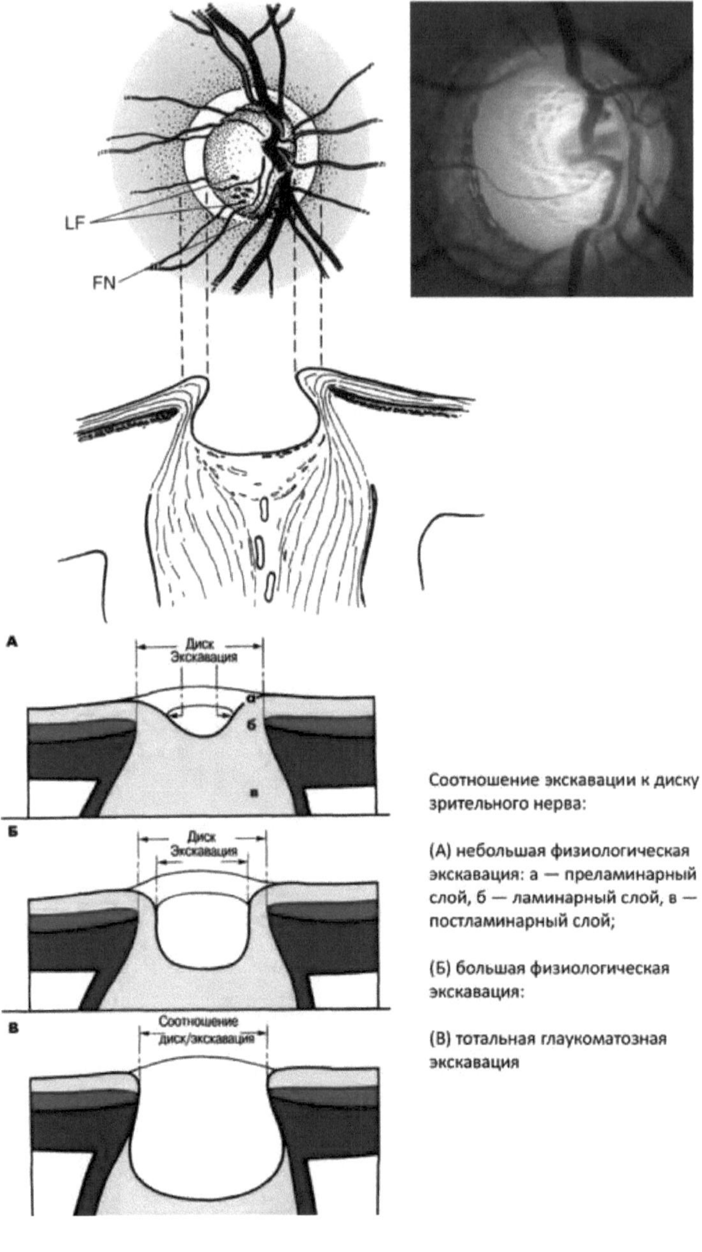

Соотношение экскавации к диску зрительного нерва:

(А) небольшая физиологическая экскавация: а — преламинарный слой, б — ламинарный слой, в — постламинарный слой;

(Б) большая физиологическая экскавация:

(В) тотальная глаукоматозная экскавация

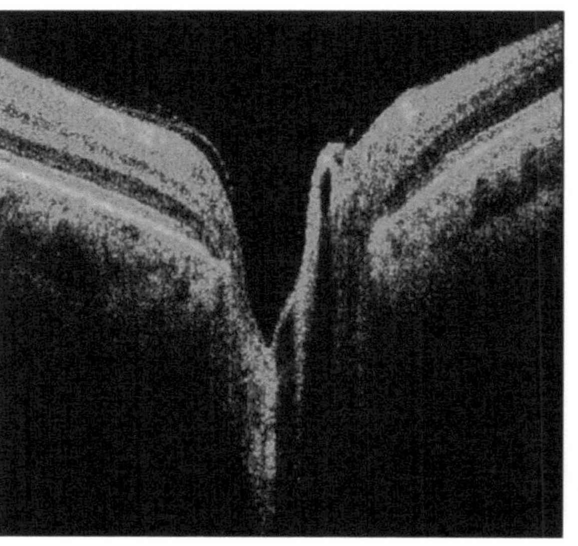

Нормальная (физиологическая экскавация ДЗН)

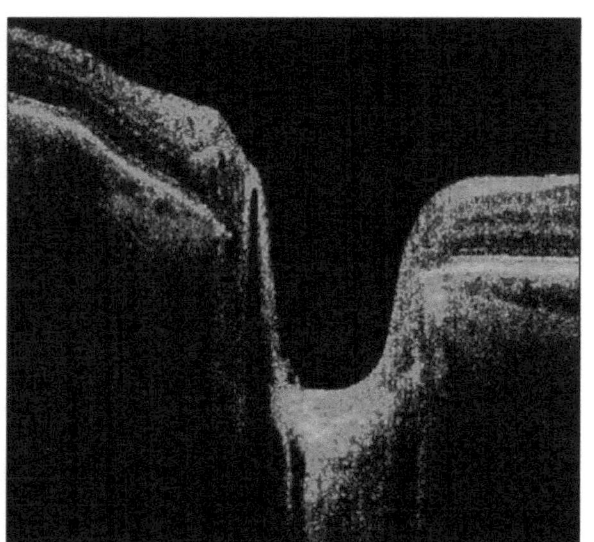

Глаукоматозная экскавация ДЗН

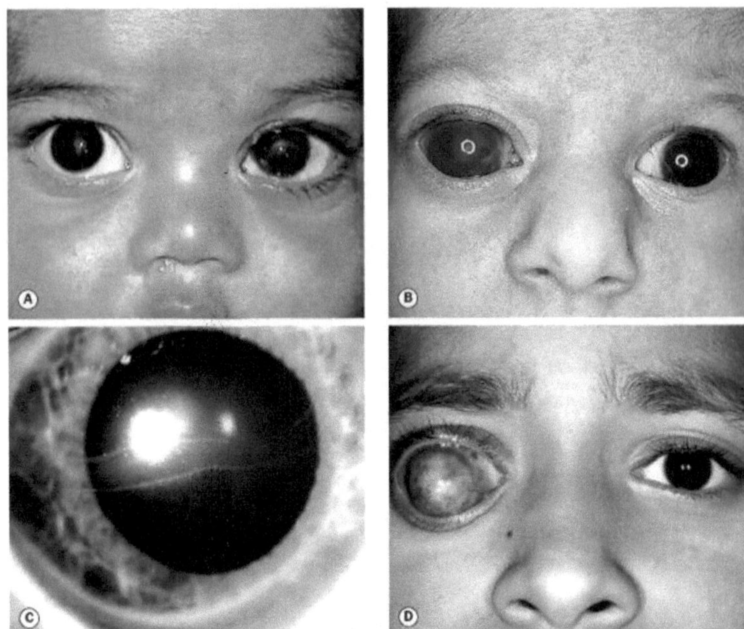

Три основных размера диска зрительного нерва в зависимости от площади:

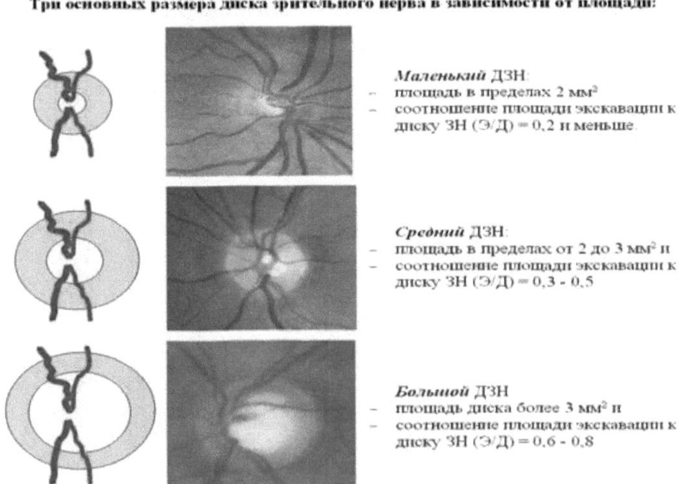

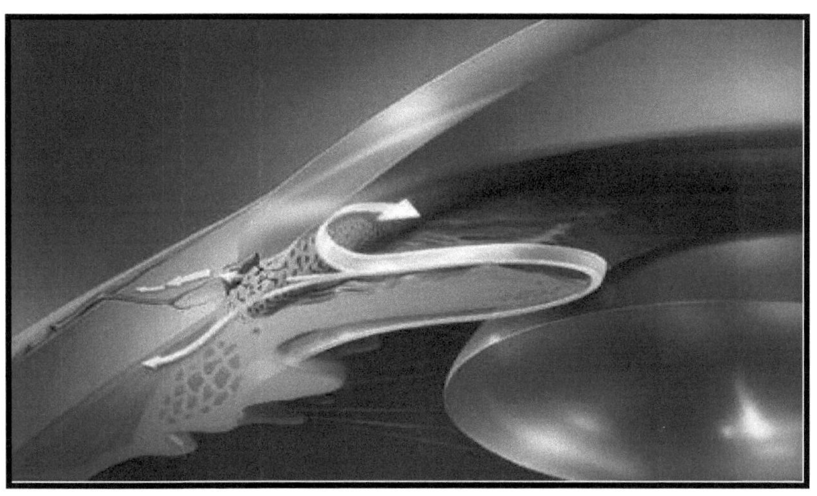

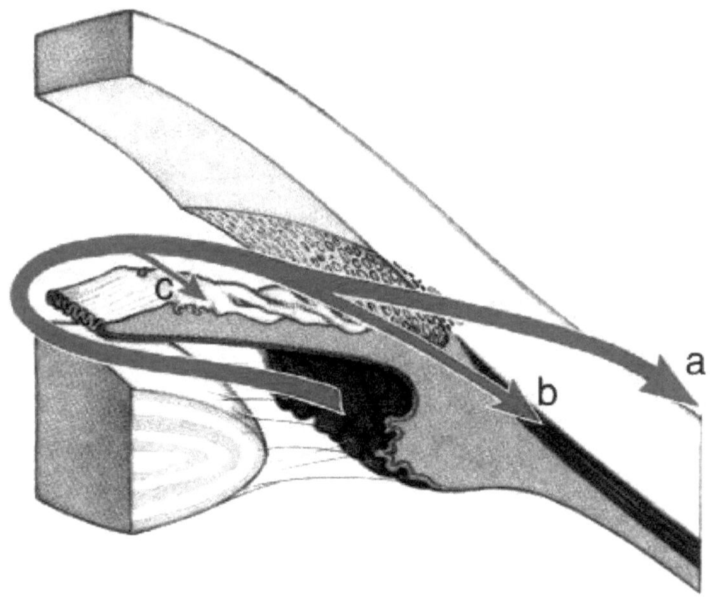

Hydrodynamics of the eye
Pathways of outflow of intraocular moisture:
a) transtrabecular; b) uveoscleral

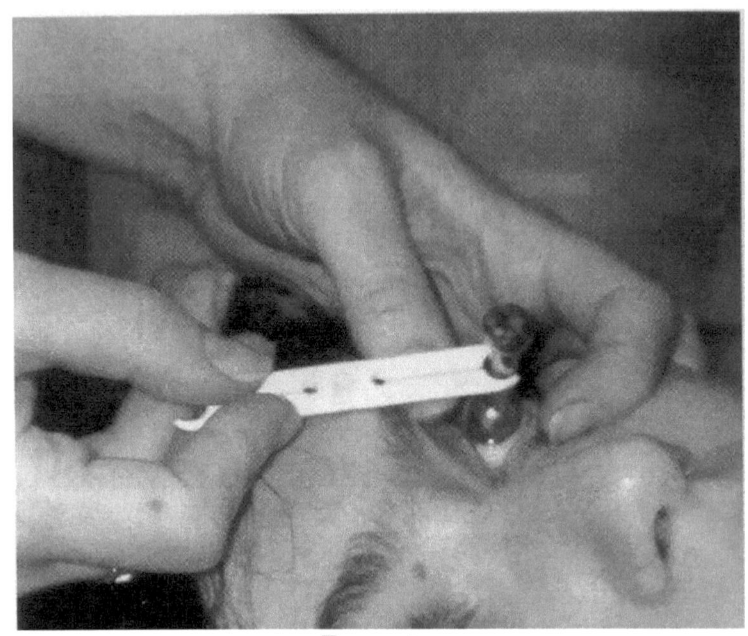

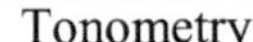
Tonometry

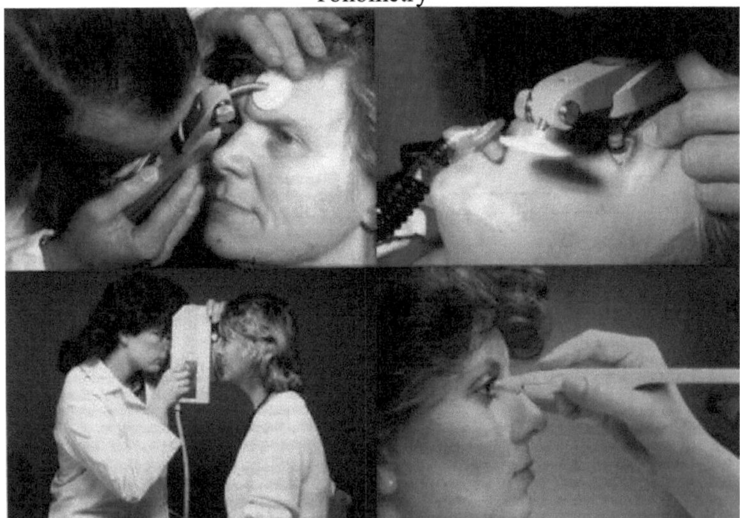

Tonometry

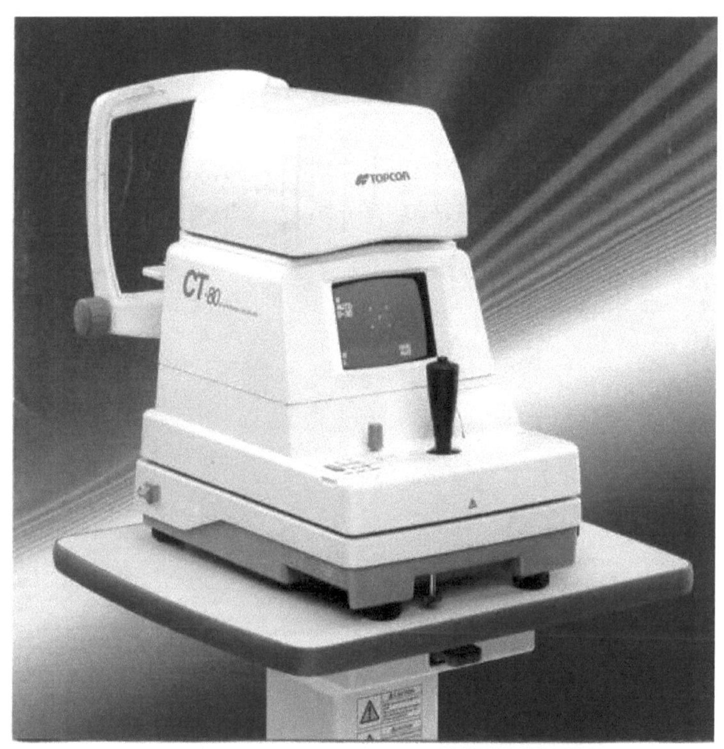

Pneumotonometer

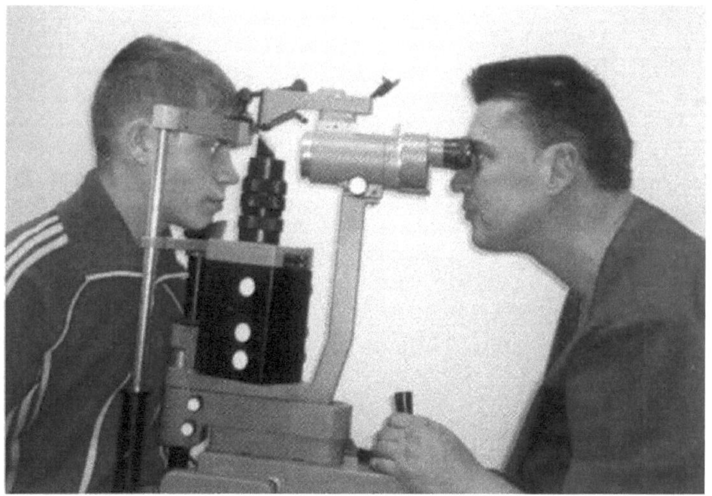

Biomicroscopy

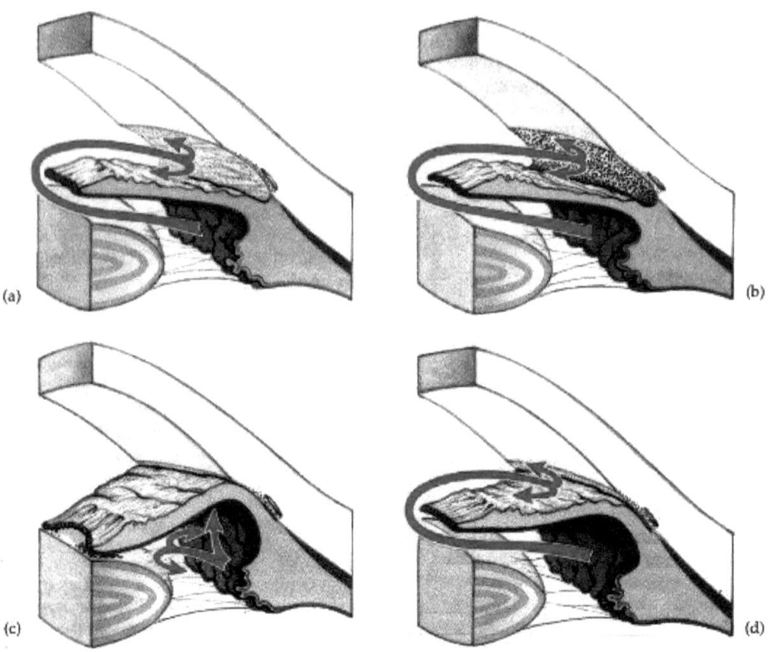

Hydrodynamic blocks: a) Schlemm's canal block; b) Trabecular block; c) Pupillary block; d) Iris base block.

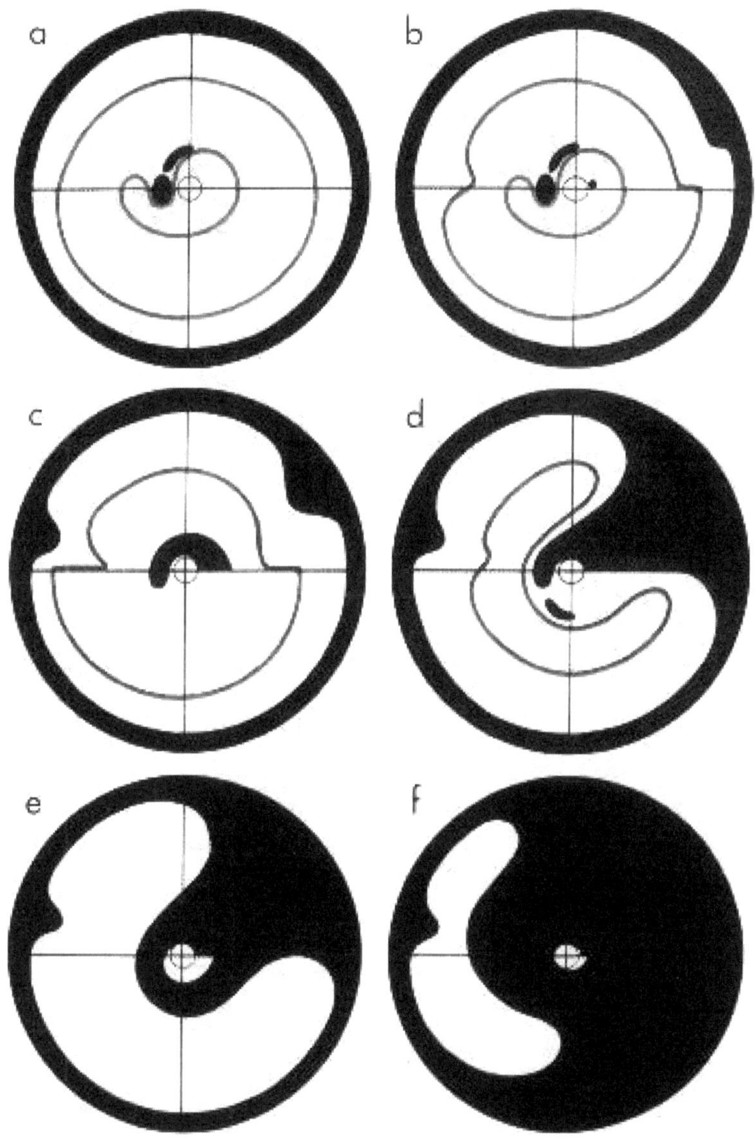

Perimetry

Changes in visual field in different stages of glaucoma

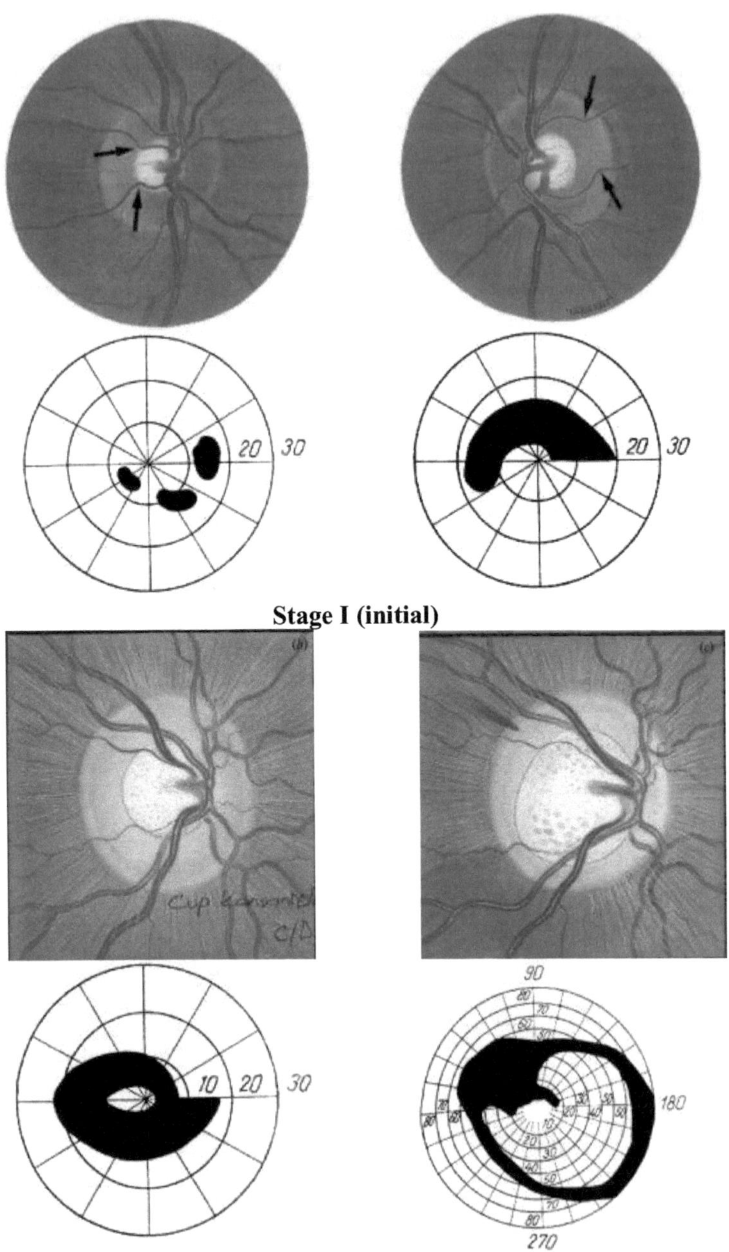

Stage I (initial)

Stage II (developed)

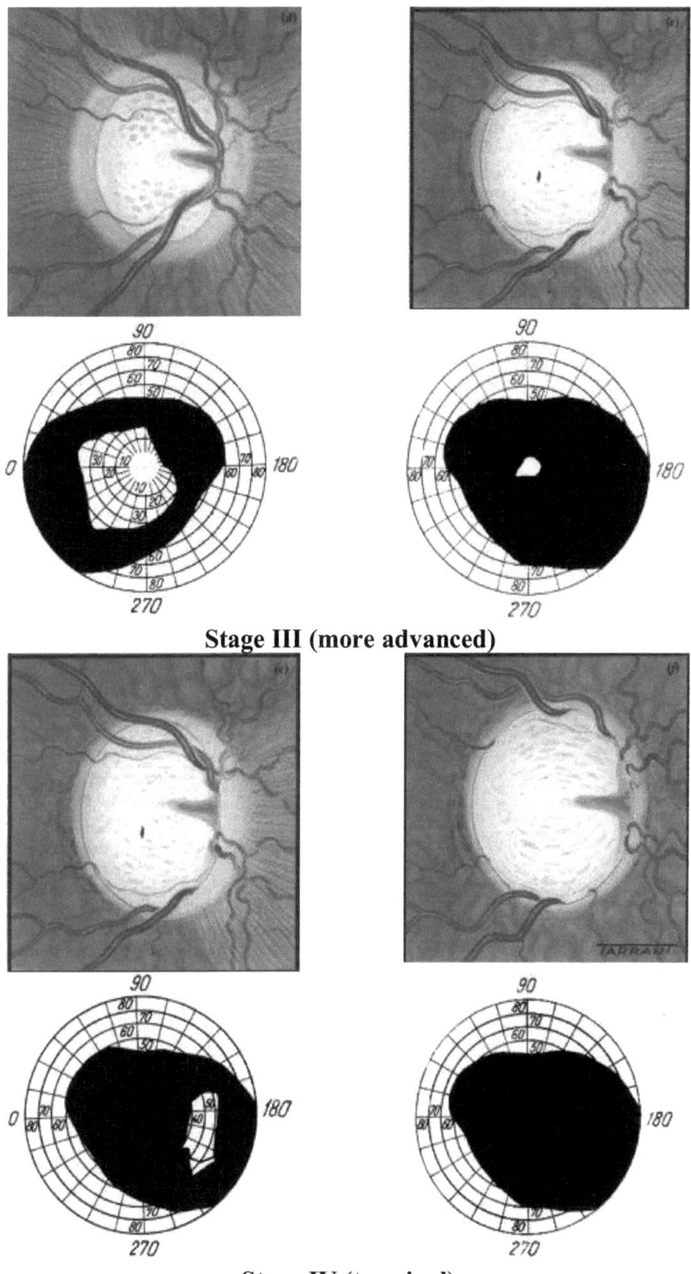

Stage III (more advanced)

Stage IV (terminal)

Phacogenic glaucoma

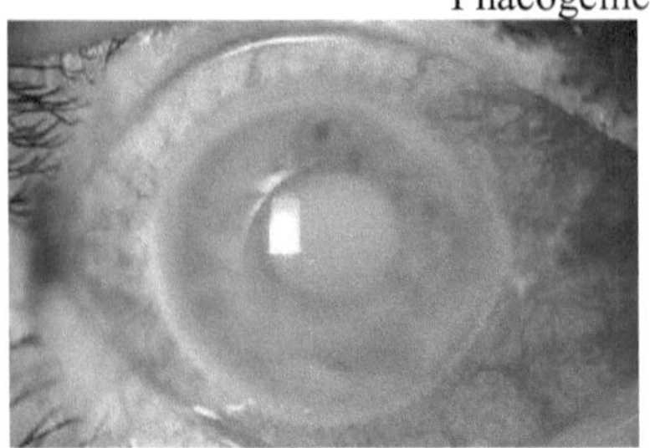

Phacomorphic

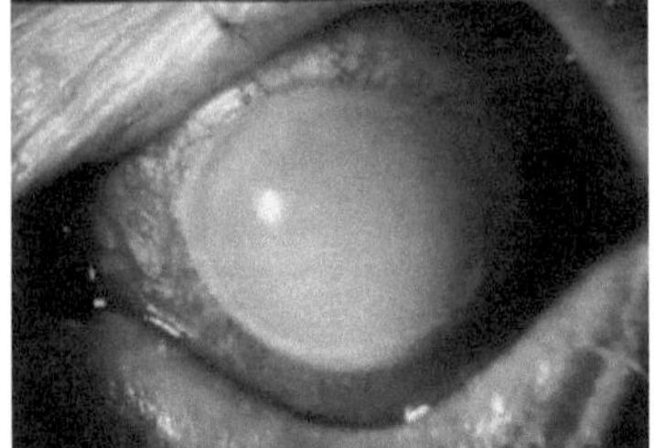

Phacolytic

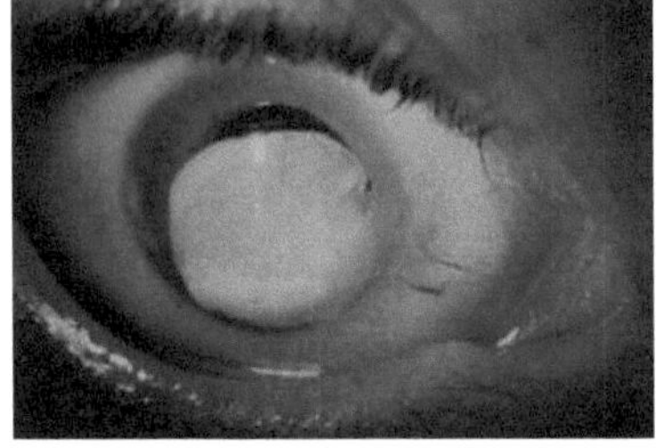

Phacotopic

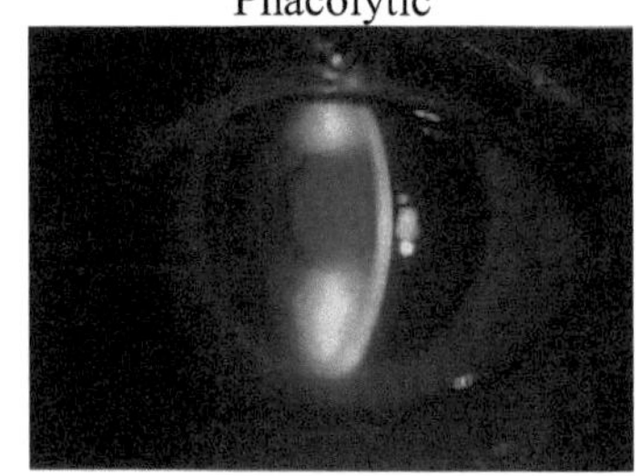

The anterior segment of the eye in cataracts

Secondary glaucomas. Vascular glaucoma.

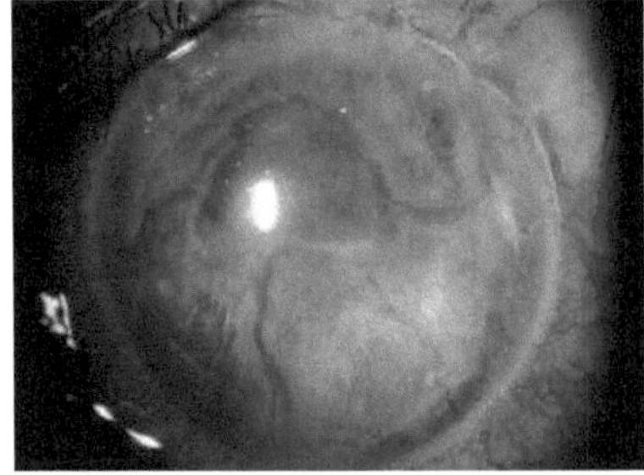

Neovascular

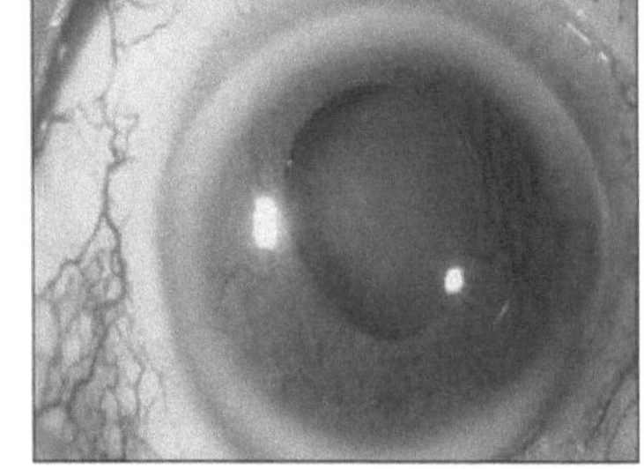

Phlebohypertensive

Secondary glaucomas. ***Dystrophic glaucoma.***

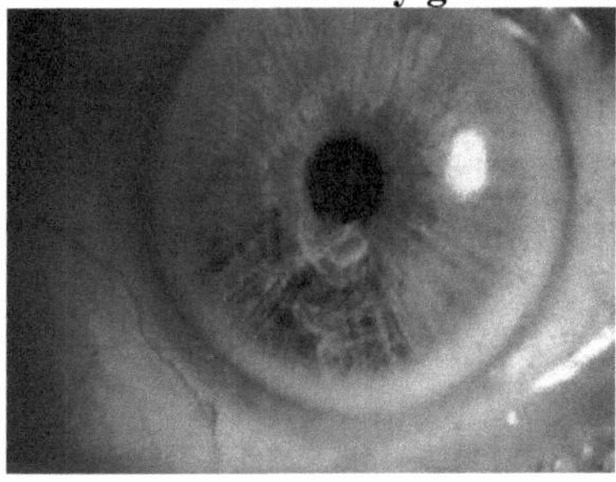

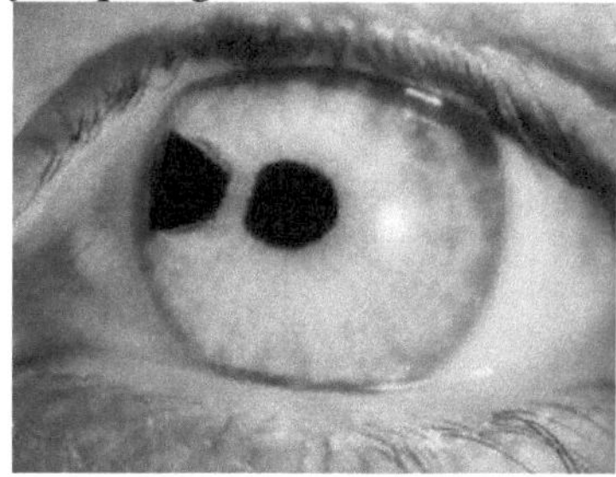

Secondary glaucomas. ***Dystrophic glaucoma.***

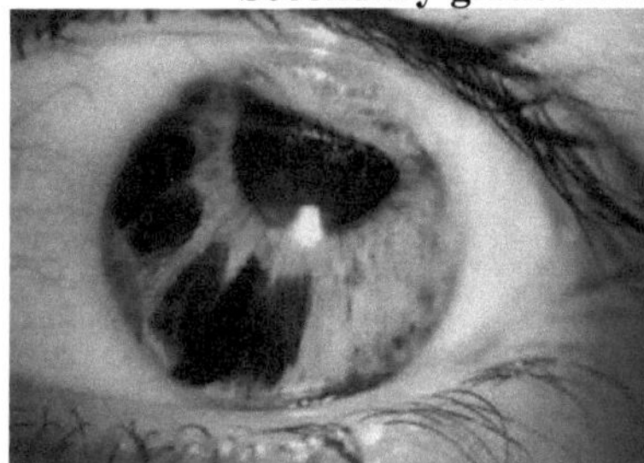

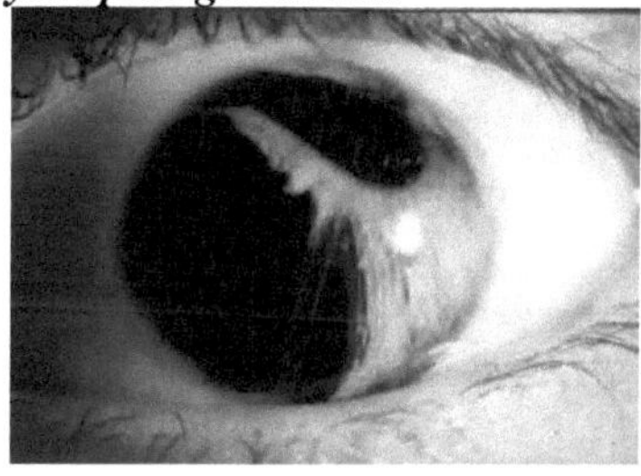

Secondary glaucoma. ***Post-traumatic glaucoma.***

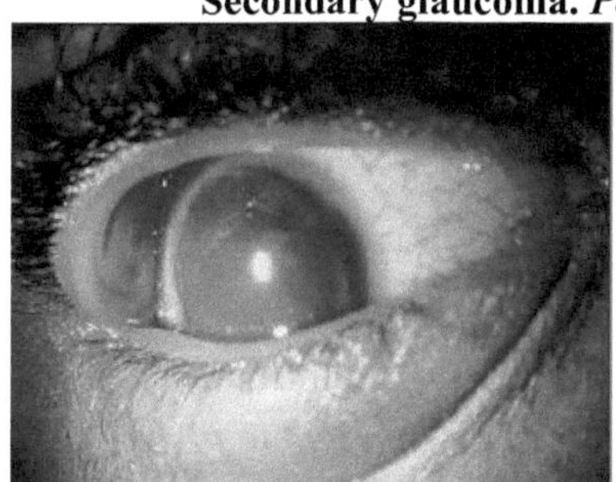

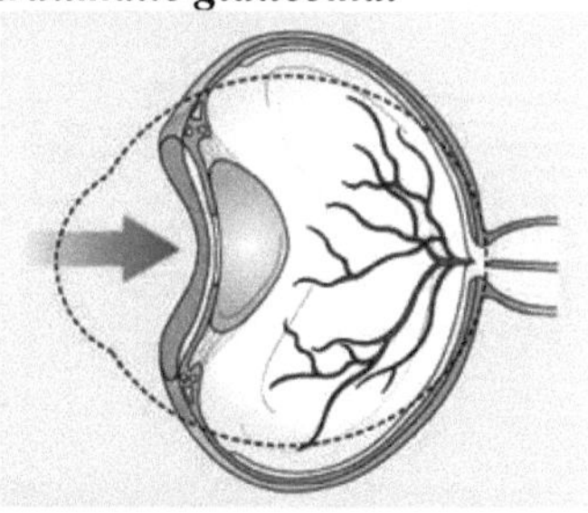

Secondary glaucomas. ***Neoplastic glaucoma***

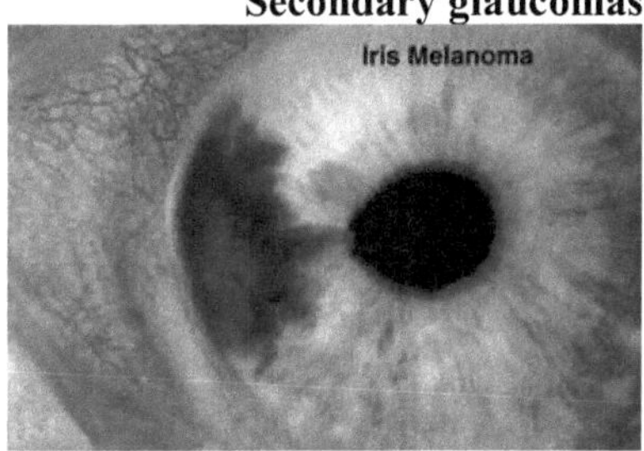

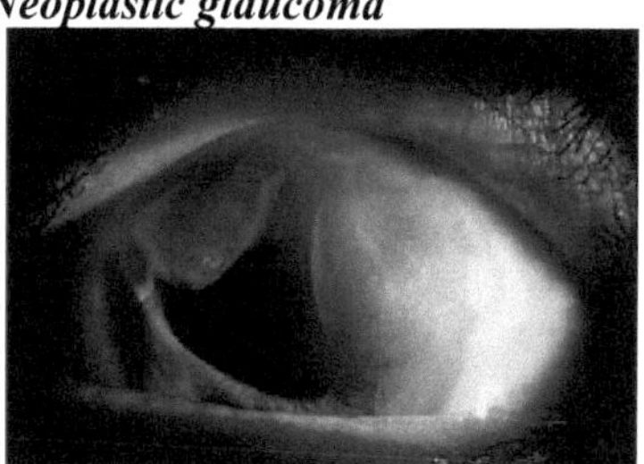

Primary congenital **glaucoma**

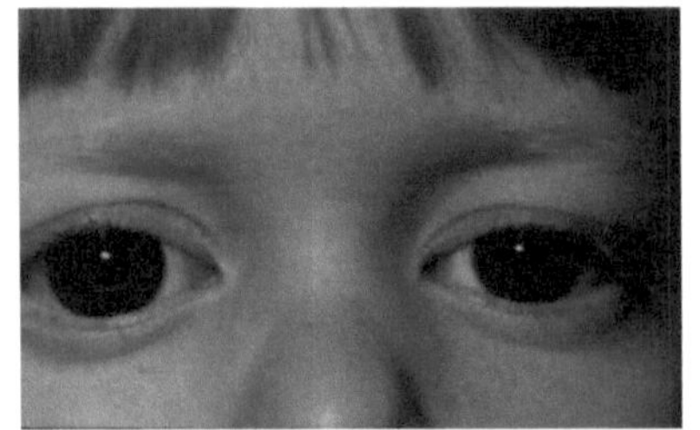

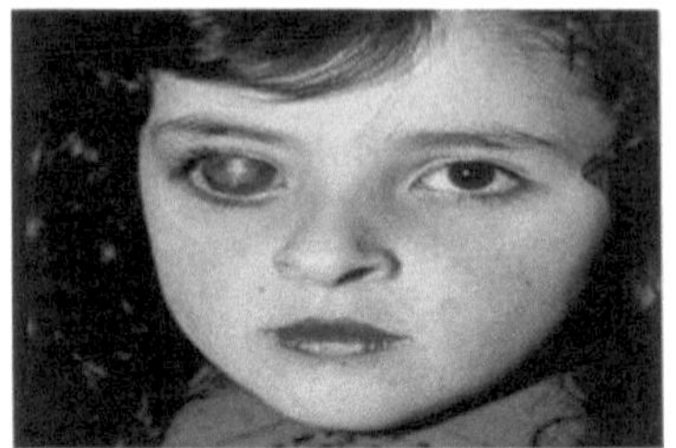

Conjoint congenital glaucoma

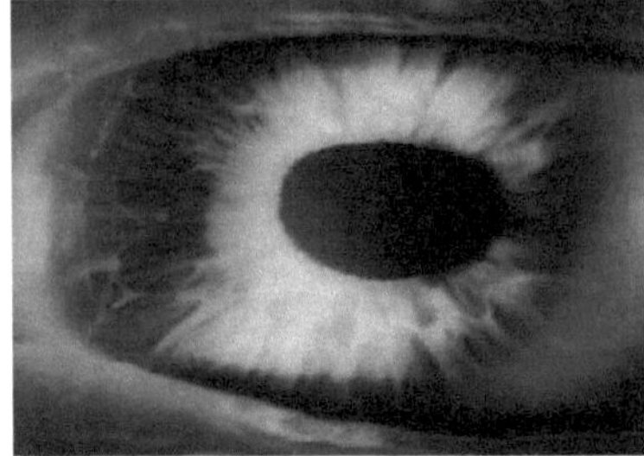

Axenfeld anomaly

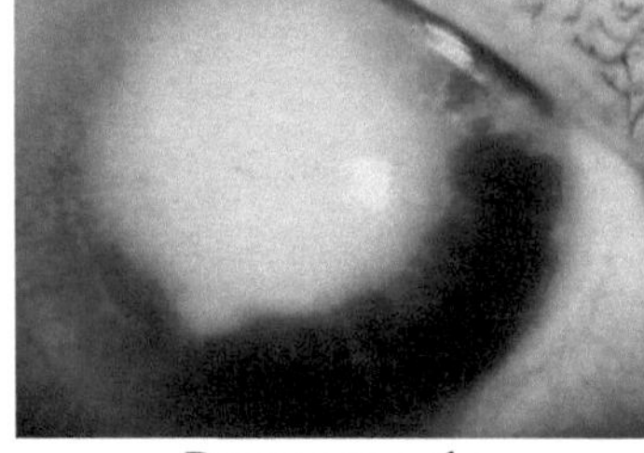

Peters anomaly

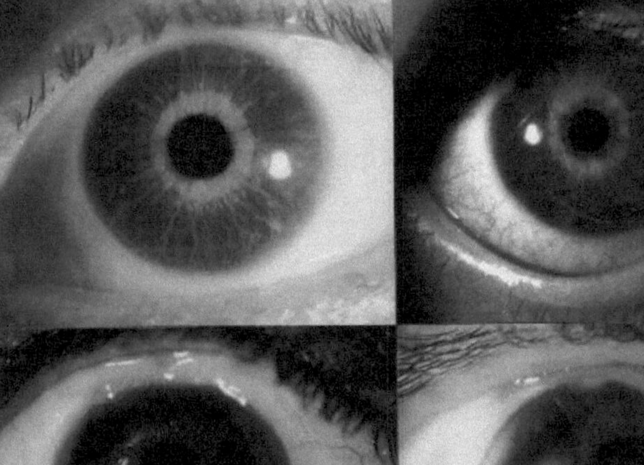

Rieger anomaly

Surgical treatment for glaucoma

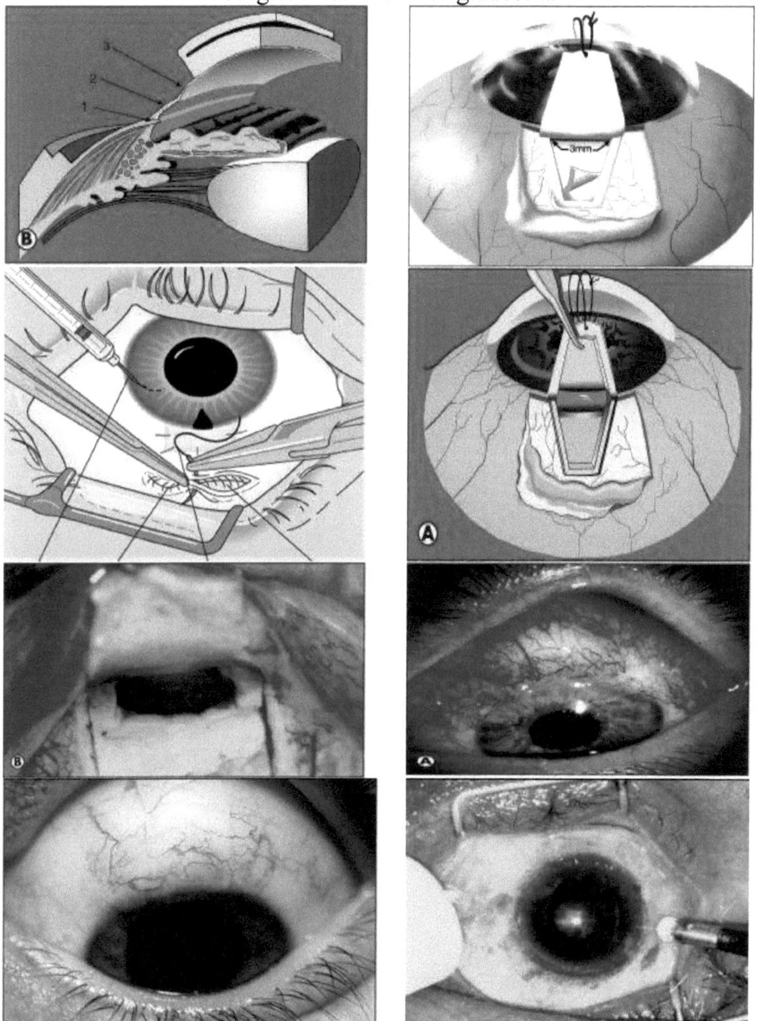

Acute onset of glaucoma

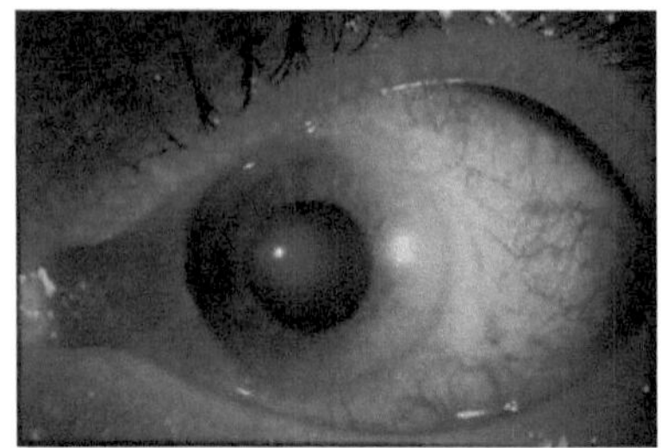

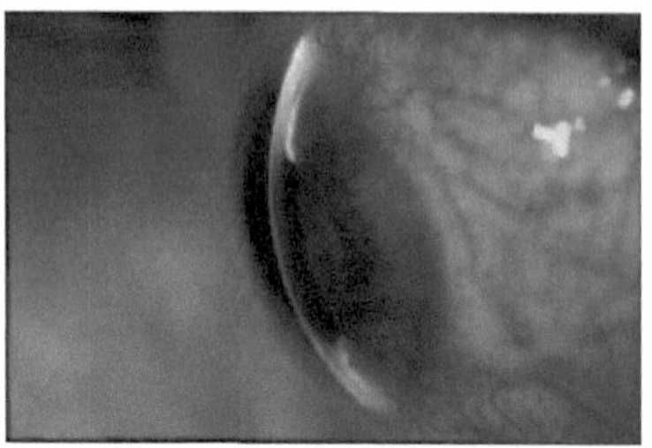

(имя и фамилия)

КРОССВОРД

Разгадай кроссворд.

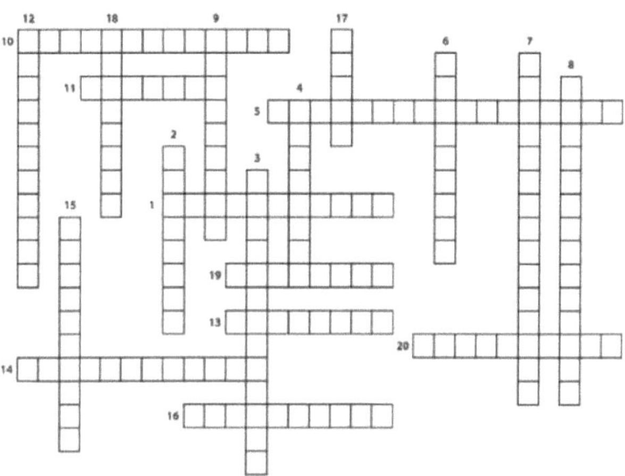

По горизонтали: 1. Показатель внутриглазного давления, который представляет собой ВГД в определенном диапазоне, характерном для индивидуума, которое является безопасным только для него, но может быть опасно для других.. 5. Каково общее название блока зрачка, стекловидного тела, трабекулярной блокады и блокады шлеммова канала?. 10. Процедура создания искусственных путей для оттока жидкости из угла передней камеры.
11. Абсолютный или относительный дефект поля зрения.
13. Основной симптом врожденной глаукомы. 14. На каком стадии глаукомы наблюдается картина поля зрения в виде «острова, окруженного морем тьмы»?. 16. Тип врожденной глаукомы, который развивается в возрасте 11-34 лет. Часто наблюдается вместе с миопической рефракцией.. 19. Объем этой камеры, являющейся основным резервуаром внутриглазной жидкости, составляет 150-250 мм3.. 20. Тип глаукомы, возникающий в результате трения пигментированного эпителия радужки о цинновы связки каждый раз в результате расширения и сужения зрачка..

По вертикали: 2. Симптом, при котором после поворота кровеносных сосудов у края диска они идут вниз по ходу экскавации и поворачиваются на дне экскавации..
3. Внутриглазная жидкость поступает в Шлеммов канал, а затем выходит из глаза по эписклеральным венам. Описание соответствует ……. 4. Какое внутриглазное давление измеряется 5-граммовым тонометрическим грузом без давления на веко?. 6. При этом типе блока затрудняется переход жидкости из задней камеры в переднюю, и избыток жидкости заставляет радужку выпячиваться вперед и перекрывать угол передней камеры.. 7. Внутриглазная жидкость проходит через цилиарное тело в супрахориоидальное пространство, а оттуда выходит из глаза через цилиарное тело, склеру и хориоидальную венозную систему. Описание соответствует ……. 8. При данном виде глаукомы амилоидоподобный фибриллярный белок скапливается на задней поверхности цилиарного тела, радужке, на поверхности передней капсулы хрусталика и в углу передней камеры.. 9. Система отверстий, напоминающая многоячеистую комнату. 12. Метод оценки угла передней камеры. 15. Этот препарат сужает зрачок, расширяет угол передней камеры и снижает внутриглазное давление за счет расширения венозных сосудов..
17. Симптом, обусловленный расширением передних артерий цилиарного тела и их врастанием в склеру в результате повышения внутриглазного давления?. 18. Какая форма глаукомы обозначается термином «тихий убийца»?.

____

(имя и фамилия)

ОТВЕТЫ

КРОССВОРД

Across:
- 1 толерантное
- 5 гидродинамический
- 10 гониопунктура
- 11 скатома
- 13 буфтальм
- 14 терминальная
- 16 ювенильная
- 19 передний
- 20 пигментная

Down:
- 2 эстакада
- 3 трабекулярный
- 4 истинно
- 6 зрачковый
- 7 увеосклеральный
- 8 эксфолиативная
- 9 трабекула
- 12 гониоскопия
- 15 пилокарпин
- 17 кобра
- 18 открытий

По горизонтали: 1. Показатель внутриглазного давления, который представляет собой ВГД в определенном диапазоне, характерном для индивидуума, которое является безопасным только для него, но может быть опасно для других.. 5. Каково общее название блока зрачка, стекловидного тела, трабекулярной блокады и блокады шлеммова канала?. 10. Процедура создания искусственных путей для оттока жидкости из угла передней камеры. 11. Абсолютный или относительный дефект поля зрения. 13. Основной симптом врожденной глаукомы. 14. На каком стадии глаукомы наблюдается картина поля зрения в виде «острова, окруженного морем тьмы»?. 16. Тип врожденной глаукомы, который развивается в возрасте 11-34 лет. Часто наблюдается вместе с миопической рефракцией.. 19. Объем этой камеры, являющейся основным резервуаром внутриглазной жидкости, составляет 150-250 мм3.. 20. Тип глаукомы, возникающий в результате трения пигментированного эпителия радужки о цинновы связки каждый раз в результате расширения и сужения зрачка..

По вертикали: 2. Симптом, при котором после поворота кровеносных сосудов у края диска они идут вниз по ходу экскавации и поворачиваются на дне экскавации..
3. Внутриглазная жидкость поступает в Шлеммов канал, а затем выходит из глаза по эписклеральным венам. Описание соответствует ……. 4. Какое внутриглазное давление измеряется 5-граммовым тонометрическим грузом без давления на веко?. 6. При этом типе блока затрудняется переход жидкости из задней камеры в переднюю, и избыток жидкости заставляет радужку выпячиваться вперед и перекрывать угол передней камеры.. 7. Внутриглазная жидкость проходит через цилиарное тело в супрахориоидальное пространство, а оттуда выходит из глаза через цилиарное тело, склеру и хориоидальную венозную систему. Описание соответствует ……. 8. При данном виде глаукомы амилоидоподобный фибриллярный белок скапливается на задней поверхности цилиарного тела, радужке, на поверхности передней капсулы хрусталика и в углу передней камеры.. 9. Система отверстий, напоминающая многоячеистую комнату. 12. Метод оценки угла передней камеры. 15. Этот препарат сужает зрачок, расширяет угол передней камеры и снижает внутриглазное давление за счет расширения венозных сосудов.. 17. Симптом, обусловленный расширением передних артерий цилиарного тела и их врастанием в склеру в результате повышения внутриглазного давления?. 18. Какая форма глаукомы обозначается термином «тихий убийца»?.

(имя и фамилия)

КРОССВОРД

Разгадай кроссворд.

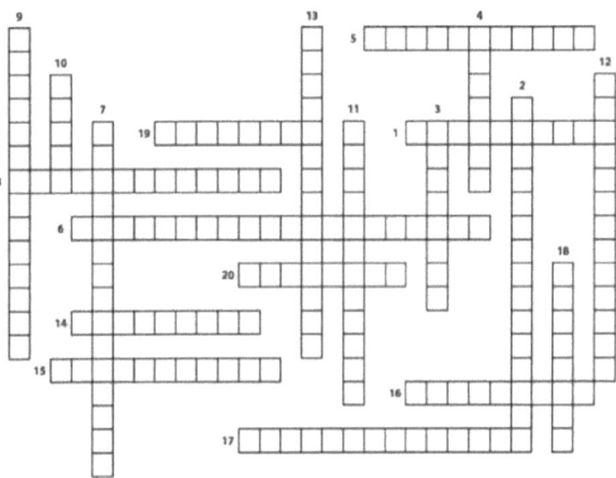

По горизонтали: 1. Этот препарат сужает зрачок, расширяет угол передней камеры и снижает внутриглазное давление за счет расширения венозных сосудов.. 5. Метод оценки угла передней камеры. 6. Тип вторичной глаукомы, при котором в глазу образуются белые сгустки фибриллярного материала. 8. Внутриглазная жидкость поступает в Шлеммов канал, а затем выходит из глаза по эписклеральным венам. Описание соответствует ……. 14. При этом типе блока затрудняется переход жидкости из задней камеры в переднюю, и избыток жидкости заставляет радужку выпячиваться вперед и перекрывать угол передней камеры.. 15. Показатель внутриглазного давления, который представляет собой ВГД в определенном диапазоне, характерном для индивидуума, которое является безопасным только для него, но может быть опасно для других.. 16. Система отверстий, напоминающая многоячеистую комнату. 17. Тип вторичной глаукомы, развивающийся при сублюксации или люксации хрусталика.. 19. Симптом, при котором после поворота кровеносных сосудов у края диска они идут вниз по ходу экскавации и поворачиваются на дне экскавации.. 20. Какая форма глаукомы обозначается термином «тихий убийца»?.

По вертикали: 2. Тип глаукомы, возникающий в результате роста волокон хрусталика при неполной или незрелой катаракте.. 3. Какое внутриглазное давление измеряется 5-граммовым тонометрическим грузом без давления на веко?. 4. Абсолютный или относительный дефект поля зрения. 7. Внутриглазная жидкость проходит через цилиарное тело в супрахориоидальное пространство, а оттуда выходит из глаза через цилиарное тело, склеру и хориоидальную венозную систему. Описание соответствует ……. 9. Тип вторичной глаукомы, развивающийся при маляции тканей хрусталика при перезрелой катаракте.. 10. Симптом, обусловленный расширением передних артерий цилиарного тела и их врастанием в склеру в результате повышения внутриглазного давления?. 11. К данному виду глаукомы относятся неоваскулярная, афакическая, ювенильная, первичная и вторичная глаукомы. После первой операции внутриглазное давление вновь повышается за счет фиброза искусственно созданных каналов оттока внутриглазной жидкости.. 12. Процедура создания искусственных путей для оттока жидкости из угла передней камеры. 13. Разновидность глаукомы, развивающаяся как осложнение гипоксических заболеваний сетчатки. Связана с такими патологиями как пролиферативная диабетическая ретинопатия и ишемическая форма окклюзии центральной вены сетчатки.. 18. Основной симптом врожденной глаукомы.

____
(имя и фамилия)

ОТВЕТЫ

КРОССВОРД

По горизонтали:
1. пилокарпин
5. гониоскопия
6. псевдоэксфолиативная
8. трабекулярный
14. зрачковый
15. толерантное
16. трабекула
17. факотопическая
19. эстакада
20. открытий

По вертикали:
2. факоморфическая
3. истинное
4. скатома
7. увеосклеральный
9. факолитическая
10. кобра
11. рефрактерная
12. гониопунктура
13. неоваскулярная
18. буфтальм

По горизонтали: 1. Этот препарат сужает зрачок, расширяет угол передней камеры и снижает внутриглазное давление за счет расширения венозных сосудов.. 5. Метод оценки угла передней камеры. 6. Тип вторичной глаукомы, при котором в глазу образуются белые сгустки фибриллярного материала. 8. Внутриглазная жидкость поступает в Шлеммов канал, а затем выходит из глаза по эписклеральным венам. Описание соответствует …….
14. При этом типе блока затрудняется переход жидкости из задней камеры в переднюю, и избыток жидкости заставляет радужку выпячиваться вперед и перекрывать угол передней камеры.. 15. Показатель внутриглазного давления, который представляет собой ВГД в определенном диапазоне, характерном для индивидуума, которое является безопасным только для него, но может быть опасно для других.. 16. Система отверстий, напоминающая многоячеистую комнату. 17. Тип вторичной глаукомы, развивающийся при сублюксации или люксации хрусталика.. 19. Симптом, при котором после поворота кровеносных сосудов у края диска они идут вниз по ходу экскавации и поворачиваются на дне экскавации.. 20. Какая форма глаукомы обозначается термином «тихий убийца»?.

По вертикали: 2. Тип глаукомы, возникающий в результате роста волокон хрусталика при неполной или незрелой катаракте.. 3. Какое внутриглазное давление измеряется 5-граммовым тонометрическим грузом без давления на веко?. 4. Абсолютный или относительный дефект поля зрения. 7. Внутриглазная жидкость проходит через цилиарное тело в супрахориоидальное пространство, а оттуда выходит из глаза через цилиарное тело, склеру и хориоидальную венозную систему. Описание соответствует
9. Тип вторичной глаукомы, развивающийся при маляции тканей хрусталика при перезрелой катаракте..
10. Симптом, обусловленный расширением передних артерий цилиарного тела и их врастанием в склеру в результате повышения внутриглазного давления?. 11. К данному виду глаукомы относятся неоваскулярная, афакическая, ювенильная, первичная и вторичная глаукомы. После первой операции внутриглазное давление вновь повышается за счет фиброза искусственно созданных каналов оттока внутриглазной жидкости.. 12. Процедура создания искусственных путей для оттока жидкости из угла передней камеры. 13. Разновидность глаукомы, развивающаяся как осложнение гипоксических заболеваний сетчатки. Связана с такими патологиями как пролиферативная диабетическая ретинопатия и ишемическая форма окклюзии центральной вены сетчатки..
18. Основной симптом врожденной глаукомы.

____

(имя и фамилия)

НАЙДИ СЛОВА

Найди и обведи **13 слов** головоломки.

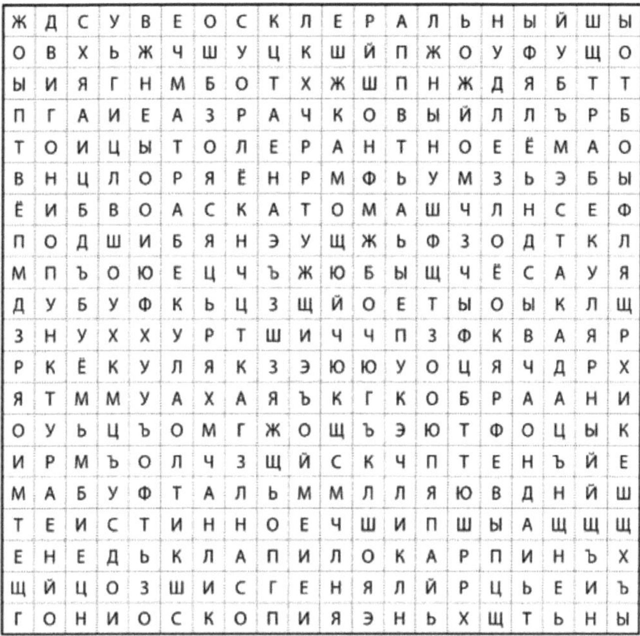

Ж	Д	С	У	В	Е	О	С	К	Л	Е	Р	А	Л	Ь	Н	Ы	Й	Ш	Ы
О	В	Х	Ь	Ж	Ч	Ш	У	Ц	К	Ш	Й	П	Ж	О	У	Ф	У	Щ	О
Ы	И	Я	Г	Н	М	Б	О	Т	Х	Ж	Ш	П	Н	Ж	Д	Я	Б	Т	Т
П	Г	А	И	Е	А	З	Р	А	Ч	К	О	В	Ы	Й	Л	Л	Ъ	Р	Б
Т	О	И	Ц	Ы	Т	О	Л	Е	Р	А	Н	Т	Н	О	Е	Ё	М	А	О
В	Н	Ц	Л	О	Р	Я	Ё	Н	Р	М	Ф	Ь	У	М	З	Ь	Э	Б	Ы
Ё	И	Б	В	О	А	С	К	А	Т	О	М	А	Ш	Ч	Л	Н	С	Е	Ф
П	О	Д	Ш	И	Б	Я	Н	Э	У	Щ	Ж	Ь	Ф	З	О	Д	Т	К	Л
М	П	Ъ	О	Ю	Е	Ц	Ч	Ъ	Ж	Ю	Б	Ы	Щ	Ч	Ё	С	А	У	Я
Д	У	Б	У	Ф	К	Ь	Ц	З	Щ	Й	О	Е	Т	Ы	О	Ы	К	Л	Щ
З	Н	У	Х	Х	У	Р	Т	Ш	И	Ч	Ч	П	З	Ф	К	В	А	Я	Р
Р	К	Ё	К	У	Л	Я	К	З	Э	Ю	Ю	У	О	Ц	Я	Ч	Д	Р	Х
Я	Т	М	М	У	А	Х	А	Я	Ъ	К	Г	К	О	Б	Р	А	А	Н	И
О	У	Ь	Ц	Ъ	О	М	Г	Ж	О	Щ	Ъ	Э	Ю	Т	Ф	О	Ц	Ы	К
И	Р	М	Ъ	О	Л	Ч	З	Щ	Й	С	К	Ч	П	Т	Е	Н	Ъ	Й	Е
М	А	Б	У	Ф	Т	А	Л	Ь	М	М	Л	Л	Я	Ю	В	Д	Н	Й	Ш
Т	Е	И	С	Т	И	Н	Н	О	Е	Ч	Ш	И	П	Ш	Ы	А	Щ	Щ	Щ
Е	Н	Е	Д	Ь	К	Л	А	П	И	Л	О	К	А	Р	П	И	Н	Ъ	Х
Щ	Й	Ц	О	З	Ш	И	С	Г	Е	Н	Я	Л	Й	Р	Ц	Ь	Е	И	Ъ
Г	О	Н	И	О	С	К	О	П	И	Я	Э	Н	Ь	Х	Щ	Т	Ь	Н	Ы

СПИСОК СЛОВ: ТРАБЕКУЛА • ИСТИННОЕ • БУФТАЛЬМ • ГОНИОПУНКТУРА • КОБРА • ЗРАЧКОВЫЙ • ПИЛОКАРПИН • УВЕОСКЛЕРАЛЬНЫЙ • ТРАБЕКУЛЯРНЫЙ • ГОНИОСКОПИЯ • ЭСТАКАДА • СКАТОМА • ТОЛЕРАНТНОЕ **(13)**

(имя и фамилия)

ОТВЕТЫ

НАЙДИ СЛОВА

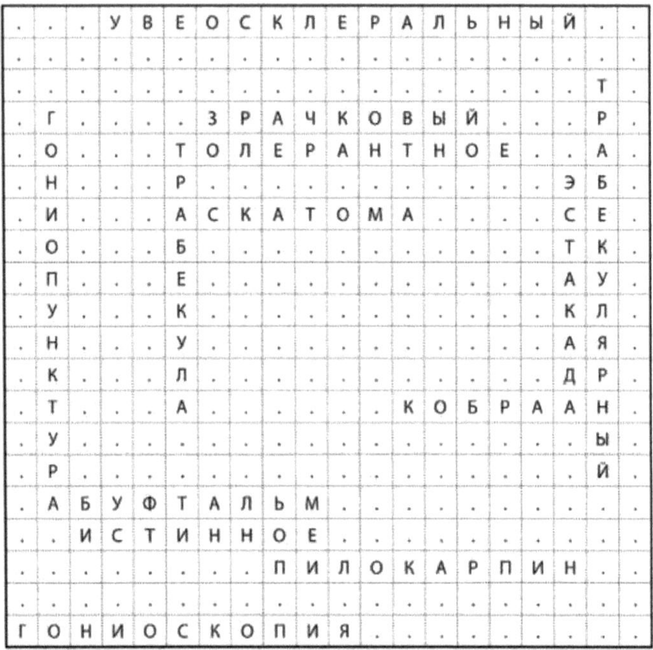

.	.	.	У	В	Е	О	С	К	Л	Е	Р	А	Л	Ь	Н	Ы	Й	.	.
.	.	.	.	.	.	.	.	.	.	.	.	.	.	.	.	.	.	.	.
.	.	.	.	.	.	.	.	.	.	.	.	.	.	.	.	.	.	Т	.
.	Г	.	.	.	.	З	Р	А	Ч	К	О	В	Ы	Й	.	.	.	Р	.
.	О	.	.	.	Т	О	Л	Е	Р	А	Н	Т	Н	О	Е	.	.	А	.
.	Н	.	.	.	Р	.	.	.	.	.	.	.	.	.	.	.	Э	Б	.
.	И	.	.	.	А	С	К	А	Т	О	М	А	.	.	.	.	С	Е	.
.	О	.	.	.	Б	.	.	.	.	.	.	.	.	.	.	.	Т	К	.
.	П	.	.	.	Е	.	.	.	.	.	.	.	.	.	.	.	А	У	.
.	У	.	.	.	К	.	.	.	.	.	.	.	.	.	.	.	К	Л	.
.	Н	.	.	.	У	.	.	.	.	.	.	.	.	.	.	.	А	Я	.
.	К	.	.	.	Л	.	.	.	.	.	.	.	.	.	.	.	Д	Р	.
.	Т	.	.	.	А	.	.	.	.	.	.	К	О	Б	Р	А	А	Н	.
.	У	.	.	.	.	.	.	.	.	.	.	.	.	.	.	.	.	Ы	.
.	Р	.	.	.	.	.	.	.	.	.	.	.	.	.	.	.	.	Й	.
.	А	Б	У	Ф	Т	А	Л	Ь	М	.	.	.	.	.	.	.	.	.	.
.	.	И	С	Т	И	Н	Н	О	Е	.	.	.	.	.	.	.	.	.	.
.	.	.	.	.	.	.	.	П	И	Л	О	К	А	Р	П	И	Н	.	.
.	.	.	.	.	.	.	.	.	.	.	.	.	.	.	.	.	.	.	.
Г	О	Н	И	О	С	К	О	П	И	Я	.	.	.	.	.	.	.	.	.

____

(имя и фамилия)

НАЙДИ СЛОВА

Найди и обведи **13 слов** головоломки.

Ё	Н	Е	О	В	А	С	К	У	Л	Я	Р	Н	А	Я	Ё	А	Ь	О	Ф
У	Э	З	Ы	И	Ц	Л	Й	П	Э	З	Н	Ш	К	Ю	Ж	П	Т	Х	Э
Я	С	Ш	Ф	А	К	О	Л	И	Т	И	Ч	Е	С	К	А	Я	Ч	Ж	Д
Ь	Е	Й	Ь	Я	Ъ	Т	Е	Р	М	И	Н	А	Л	Ь	Н	А	Я	Д	Е
Б	А	Й	Д	Х	К	И	У	Т	Ч	П	Ш	А	Д	Т	Ж	Я	Е	Ъ	Й
М	Д	Д	Ф	А	К	О	Т	О	П	И	Ч	Е	С	К	А	Я	Б	Д	Я
А	Р	Х	Б	Ц	Н	Я	Ш	П	И	Г	М	Е	Н	Т	Н	А	Я	Ю	Щ
П	В	А	Э	К	С	Ф	О	Л	И	А	Т	И	В	Н	А	Я	У	Ы	Щ
П	Щ	Ш	А	Е	Ъ	Ч	Т	М	У	Д	Щ	Ь	У	Г	Ж	Ъ	Я	Ю	Р
А	Л	Г	И	Д	Р	О	Д	И	Н	А	М	И	Ч	Е	С	К	И	Й	Щ
Я	Ш	Э	К	Р	Л	В	Ъ	Ч	М	Ы	Х	Х	С	Ё	Ь	Ф	Х	Ч	Ч
Е	В	К	Ё	Е	Ъ	Е	Ь	Ъ	Щ	Ъ	Щ	И	С	Л	Р	Г	Н	А	Д
Г	Ф	А	К	О	М	О	Р	Ф	И	Ч	Е	С	К	А	Я	У	Т	Ч	К
Ю	И	Й	О	Б	У	Ф	Т	А	Л	Ь	М	К	М	Р	Р	М	Л	А	В
Ъ	Ш	Ж	Е	С	П	Р	М	Ш	Р	Ы	Ш	Ы	Щ	О	Ч	Я	И	У	О
П	С	Е	В	Д	О	Э	К	С	Ф	О	Л	И	А	Т	И	В	Н	А	Я
Л	Ъ	Ж	С	Ф	Г	Г	Г	Ж	З	Ш	Т	К	О	Б	Р	А	Л	А	А
Ф	Л	Ъ	Й	Ц	Е	Ъ	Р	Ч	З	М	Ф	К	П	Ж	Л	М	О	Г	Е
О	Ф	Д	Ю	В	Е	Н	И	Л	Ь	Н	А	Я	Е	У	Ь	Э	Й	Щ	Р
Ц	Ю	Ц	Б	Ё	Ъ	Р	Е	Ф	Р	А	К	Т	Е	Р	Н	А	Я	Е	Ы

СПИСОК СЛОВ: ГИДРОДИНАМИЧЕСКИЙ • ТЕРМИНАЛЬНАЯ • ЮВЕНИЛЬНАЯ • ЭКСФОЛИАТИВНАЯ • ПИГМЕНТНАЯ • РЕФРАКТЕРНАЯ • НЕОВАСКУЛЯРНАЯ • ФАКОМОРФИЧЕСКАЯ • ФАКОЛИТИЧЕСКАЯ • ФАКОТОПИЧЕСКАЯ • ПСЕВДОЭКСФОЛИАТИВНАЯ • БУФТАЛЬМ • КОБРА **(13)**

____

(имя и фамилия)

ОТВЕТЫ

НАЙДИ СЛОВА

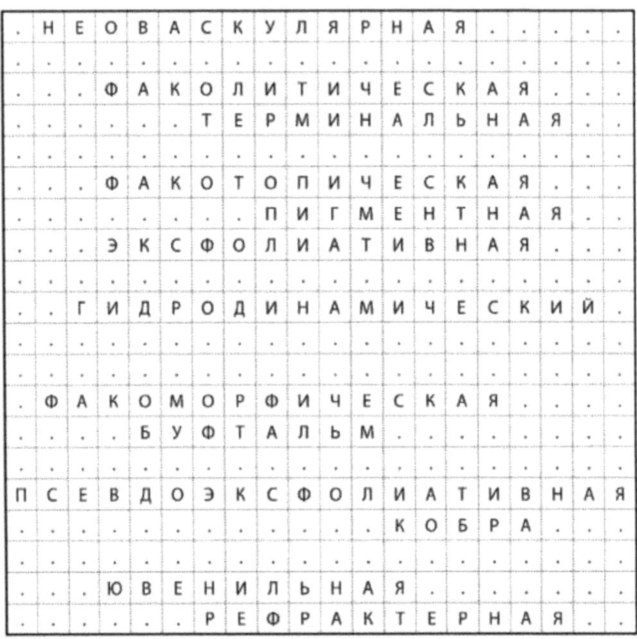

.	Н	Е	О	В	А	С	К	У	Л	Я	Р	Н	А	Я	.	.	.	.	.
.	.	.	.	.	.	.	.	.	.	.	.	.	.	.	.	.	.	.	.
.	.	.	Ф	А	К	О	Л	И	Т	И	Ч	Е	С	К	А	Я	.	.	.
.	.	.	.	.	.	Т	Е	Р	М	И	Н	А	Л	Ь	Н	А	Я	.	.
.	.	.	.	.	.	.	.	.	.	.	.	.	.	.	.	.	.	.	.
.	.	.	Ф	А	К	О	Т	О	П	И	Ч	Е	С	К	А	Я	.	.	.
.	.	.	.	.	.	.	.	П	И	Г	М	Е	Н	Т	Н	А	Я	.	.
.	.	.	Э	К	С	Ф	О	Л	И	А	Т	И	В	Н	А	Я	.	.	.
.	.	.	.	.	.	.	.	.	.	.	.	.	.	.	.	.	.	.	.
.	.	Г	И	Д	Р	О	Д	И	Н	А	М	И	Ч	Е	С	К	И	Й	.
.	.	.	.	.	.	.	.	.	.	.	.	.	.	.	.	.	.	.	.
.	.	.	.	.	.	.	.	.	.	.	.	.	.	.	.	.	.	.	.
.	Ф	А	К	О	М	О	Р	Ф	И	Ч	Е	С	К	А	Я	.	.	.	.
.	.	.	.	Б	У	Ф	Т	А	Л	Ь	М	.	.	.	.	.	.	.	.
.	.	.	.	.	.	.	.	.	.	.	.	.	.	.	.	.	.	.	.
П	С	Е	В	Д	О	Э	К	С	Ф	О	Л	И	А	Т	И	В	Н	А	Я
.	.	.	.	.	.	.	.	.	.	.	.	К	О	Б	Р	А	.	.	.
.	.	.	.	.	.	.	.	.	.	.	.	.	.	.	.	.	.	.	.
.	.	.	Ю	В	Е	Н	И	Л	Ь	Н	А	Я	.	.	.	.	.	.	.
.	.	.	.	.	.	Р	Е	Ф	Р	А	К	Т	Е	Р	Н	А	Я	.	.

Анаграмма — беспорядочная перестановка букв в слове, которая создает другое слово. Разгадайте анаграммы и запишите ответы в специально отведенном месте.

Анаграмма

Анаграммы — Ответы

1. ЛАКЕТБРУА
2. СИИЕНОТН
3. УЛАМБЬФТ
4. ТОГУУИНПОНРАК
5. ЫЙРТТИКО
6. РКОАБ
7. ЫРАКВЧЙЗО
8. ИРАПЛИКНПО
9. ЕЫЛУОЕЙКСРАВЬНЛ
10. РАРЙЛУЫНЯБКЕТ

Анаграмма. Ответы

Анаграммы — Ответы

1. ЛАКЕТБРУА
   ТРАБЕКУЛА
2. СИИЕНОТН
   ИСТИННОЕ
3. УЛАМБЬФТ
   БУФТАЛЬМ
4. ТОГУУИНПОНРАК
   ГОНИОПУНКТУРА
5. ЫЙРТТИКО
   ОТКРЫТИЙ
6. РКОАБ
   КОБРА
7. ЫРАКВЧЙЗО
   ЗРАЧКОВЫЙ
8. ИРАПЛИКНПО
   ПИЛОКАРПИН
9. ЕЫЛУОЕЙКСРАВЬНЛ
   УВЕОСКЛЕРАЛЬНЫЙ
10. РАРЙЛУЫНЯБКЕТ
   ТРАБЕКУЛЯРНЫЙ

Анаграмма — беспорядочная перестановка букв в слове, которая создает другое слово. Разгадайте анаграммы и запишите ответы в специально отведенном месте.

Анаграмма

Анаграммы — Ответы

1. МКНДГИЧДИЕИОИРАЙС
2. ЕЯНАНРЬТАИМЛ
3. НИЕВАНЯЬЮЛ
4. АКАЭОФНТИЯСИЛВ
5. НЕЯТПИГНАМ
6. ТРКЕФЕРАЯРАН
7. НЯАНЯУКВЕРЛОСА
8. ЯМИФКАЧАОЕРСОКФ
9. ЯФАОКИЧТАЛСЕКИ
10. ПАКСЧООФТИКЯАЕ

Анаграмма. Ответы

Анаграммы — Ответы

1. МКНДГИЧДИЕИОИРАЙС

   ГИДРОДИНАМИЧЕСКИЙ

2. ЕЯНАНРЬТАИМЛ

   ТЕРМИНАЛЬНАЯ

3. НИЕВАНЯЬЮЛ

   ЮВЕНИЛЬНАЯ

4. АКАЭОФНТИЯСИЛВ

   ЭКСФОЛИАТИВНАЯ

5. НЕЯТПИГНАМ

   ПИГМЕНТНАЯ

6. ТРКЕФЕРАЯРАН

   РЕФРАКТЕРНАЯ

7. НЯАНЯУКВЕРЛОСА

   НЕОВАСКУЛЯРНАЯ

8. ЯМИФКАЧАОЕРСОКФ

   ФАКОМОРФИЧЕСКАЯ

9. ЯФАОКИЧТАЛСЕКИ

   ФАКОЛИТИЧЕСКАЯ

10. ПАКСЧООФТИКЯАЕ

    ФАКОТОПИЧЕСКАЯ

LITERATURE

Basic literature:

1. Bochkareva A.A. Eye diseases: textbook / A.A. Bochkareva, T.I. Bochkareva A.A., Bochkareva T.I., Eroshevsky A.P., Nesterov A.P. et al; Ed. by A.A. Bochkareva. - Moscow: Medicine, 1989.
2. Kopaeva V.G. Eye diseases. Textbook. - Moscow. Ophthalmology. 2018 г.

Further reading:

1. Egorov E. A..Ophthalmology. Textbook. -M. GEOTAR-Media. 2018 г.
2. Sidorenko E.N. Ophthalmology. Moscow 2002.
3. Somov E.E. Clinical ophthalmology. Moscow, 2017.
4. Clinical ophthalmology. A systematic approach. J. Kanski. 9th edition. 2020.

Internet resources:

1. www.eyenews.ru
2. www.tma.uz
3. www.helmholth/eyeinstitute.ru
4. www.eyeworld.com
5. www.ziyonet.uz

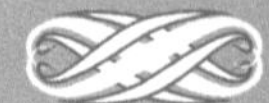

CONTENTS

INTRODUCTION 3

GLAUCOMA 5

THEORETICAL PART 9

ANALYTICAL PART 25

PRACTICAL PART 30

LITERATURE 69

CONTENTS 70

FOR IMMEDIATE RELEASE 71

FOR IMMEDIATE RELEASE

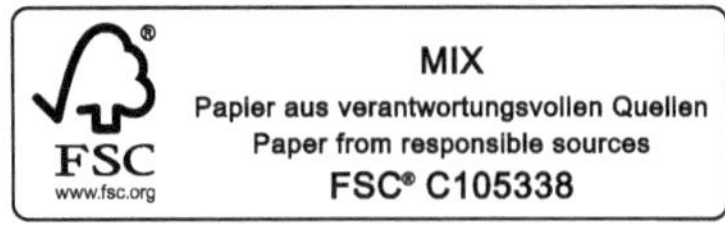

Printed by Books on Demand GmbH, Norderstedt / Germany